For Jamie

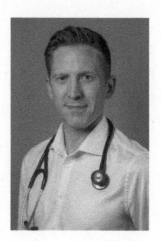

Dr Brad McKay is an Australian science communicator, TV host and GP at his clinic in Sydney. He is an experienced broadcaster, interviewer and public commentator, appearing regularly on TV and radio, including as a host of ABC's *Catalyst* and a regular commentator on *The Today Show*, and presenting several medical podcasts for health professionals. He is also on the editorial board for *The Medical Republic* magazine.

Brad has hosted the Logie-nominated *Embarrassing Bodies Down Under*, a show dedicated to decreasing stigma and raising awareness of traditionally 'taboo' health topics. He is a member of the Immunisation Coalition, and an Ambassador for the Immunisation Foundation and the Stroke Foundation.

Dr Brad McKay

FAKE
MEDICINE

Exposing the wellness crazes, cons
and quacks costing us our health

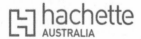

Important note to readers: Although every effort has been made to ensure the contents of this book are accurate, it must not be treated as a substitute for qualified medical advice. Always consult a qualified medical practitioner. Neither the author nor the publisher can be held responsible for any loss or claim arising out of the use, or misuse, of the suggestions made or the failure to take professional medical advice.

Pseudonyms have been used in this book and other details altered where necessary to protect the identity and privacy of people mentioned.

Quote on page 3 from Amy Remeikis reproduced with permission.
Quote on page 3 from *Please Like Me* used with permission from Pigeon Fancier Productions and John & Josh International.
Quote on page 3 from 'Storm' by Tim Minchin reproduced with permission.
Quotes on page 62 from Doctor Nikki Stamp from *Pretty Unhealthy: Why our obsession with looking healthy is making us sick* reproduced with permission.

 hachette
AUSTRALIA

Published in Australia and New Zealand in 2021
by Hachette Australia
(an imprint of Hachette Australia Pty Limited)
Level 17, 207 Kent Street, Sydney NSW 2000
www.hachette.com.au

10 9 8 7 6 5 4 3 2 1

A catalogue record for this book is available from the National Library of Australia

ISBN: 978 0 7336 4686 7 (paperback)

Cover design by Christabella Designs
Cover photograph courtesy of iStock
Author photograph courtesy of Cain Cooper
Typeset in Sabon LT Std by Kirby Jones
Printed and bound in Australia by McPherson's Printing Group

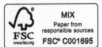

MIX
Paper from
responsible sources
FSC® C001695

The paper this book is printed on is certified against the Forest Stewardship Council® Standards. McPherson's Printing Group holds FSC® chain of custody certification SA-COC-005379. FSC® promotes environmentally responsible, socially beneficial and economically viable management of the world's forests.

CONTENTS

INTRODUCTION

Fake medicine. Fake news. Alternative facts. Fake science. Conspiracy theories.

The world is full of misinformation. It enters our lives through our television screens, our newspapers and our radio airwaves. We pass it on to one another at school pickup, in local cafes and in the workplace. And it filters through our social media feeds, slowly filling our heads with untruths and distorting our reality.

For years I have been trying to battle health falsehoods in my own little way; I've been a keyboard warrior on the socials, calling out friends, family and strangers for passing it down the line. I've appeared on television, trying to feed people the latest medical facts alongside their morning coffee and toast. And I've written articles for news outlets, trying to convince readers to think more critically about their favourite celebrity's new weight loss product.

As the host of *Embarrassing Bodies Down Under* I relished the opportunity to educate via stealth – entertaining the audience as they voyeuristically watched people undergo some pretty significant medical procedures.

But I've often thought of myself as a lone voice – the only one willing to ask Grandma to stop sharing fake flu treatments on Facebook.

This is no longer the case.

The COVID-19 pandemic has taught humanity the devastating impact the spread of misinformation can have on our health. Viral posts about the inability of masks to protect people have caused significant pain and suffering, the former American President's sarcastic suggestion of injecting bleach to kill the virus saw calls to poison centres rise across the country, and anti-vaccine activists have found new audiences.

Our modern world provides us with free and easy access to more information than ever before, and yet we as a society still haven't discovered a sure-fire way to sift fact from fiction. More needs to be done. We must be more critical. We must battle fake medicine.

'You know what they call "alternative medicine" that's been proved to work? Medicine.'

Tim Minchin, 'Storm'

'You can have alternative music, alternative fashion, alternative ideas. You can't have alternative facts. Putting the word "alternative" before "medicine" is like pointing at a dog and saying, "That's my alternative cat." It's still not a cat.'

Josh Thomas, *Please Like Me*

'I once read an analysis on conspiracy theorists, which posited that they, more than most, crave security and order. So it's easier to believe that big bad shadowy forces are in control, because that way, someone is still in control. But f**k you if you're spreading bulls**t.'

Amy Remeikis, Tweet, 8 January 2020

CHAPTER 1

A PAIN IN THE BUM

Navigating a health crisis can be a confusing and awful experience. I understand the lure of alternatives to modern medicine and have even fallen for them myself.

In fact, my journey to become a general practitioner was influenced by the confusion and misinformation I encountered as a teenage patient.

Like many fifteen-year-olds I was a pimply mess of embarrassment, hormones and deep-seated anxieties as I sat next to my mum at the local clinic. We were seeing our family doctor and were about to receive some bad advice.

I told my GP what the problem was, while the faint scent of hospital-grade antiseptic wafted up my nostrils. He paused and gazed out the window, then turned to face me, peered over his glasses and asked, 'What shall we do with you?'

He was the doctor and I was the patient, so I sincerely hoped this was a rhetorical question.

Pain was a familiar experience for me by that stage. Not the pain of teenage angst – although there was a fair bit of that too – but a physical pain in my back that my family had assumed would disappear as I got older. It hadn't.

A few years earlier, I was mucking around at school when one of my ballet friends lightly performed a *grand jeté* into my lower back. The kick wasn't that hard, but I wound up on the floor writhing in agony. Pain rippled through my body like an earthquake rolling across the landscape. I'd never experienced pain so severe in my life. It engulfed every cell of my body and reached a crescendo where my consciousness protectively departed.

My brain came back into the room when the feeling subsided and I found myself on the ground with tears in my eyes, surrounded by my friends' concerned expressions.

The pain disappeared just as quickly as it had arrived, and I didn't think much of it – but several months later it came back with a vengeance.

I'd experience the odd, sharp twinge during the daytime, but night-time was worse. Falling asleep was all right, but I'd inevitably roll onto my back and wake up in a hot, sweaty mess. My lower back ached like my buttocks had been attacked by a sizzling cattle prod.

Our family doctor looked at me quizzically and eventually deduced, 'Lower back pain is pretty normal. Eighty per cent of the population get it at some stage, in fact I've got exactly the same thing right now. Our physiotherapist will fix you up in a jiffy.'

I wasn't quite sure that back pain in a fifteen-year-old would have the same cause as back pain experienced by a 55-year-old GP, but he was the expert.

A kind-hearted physiotherapist performed an assessment. She taught me some exercises to improve my posture and attempted to massage my lower back, but it was extremely uncomfortable.

I trusted my doctor and believed him when he told me this treatment would help me get better, so I never complained about the pain. I'd grip the edge of the massage table until my knuckles turned white and every muscle in my body was contorted in agony.

When I didn't respond to treatment, my physiotherapist sent me back to see my GP. His working diagnosis was that I likely had a disc prolapse in my lumbar spine, causing sciatic pain to radiate into my buttocks, but a CT scan showed that everything was normal.

He sent me back to the physiotherapist who was happy to continue therapy, satisfied that my anatomy wasn't hiding anything sinister.

Her usual treatments clearly weren't working and my back had become too painful to touch, so she changed tack and commenced heat therapy instead.

She pulled out a handmade device that looked rather primitive – a piece of timber wrapped in carpet with electrical wires hanging out. She positioned the device over my buttocks as I lay prone on the couch.

I watched as she plugged it in, switched it on and left the room. After twenty minutes, she returned to the delightfully warm aroma of burnt carpet and found me grimacing with intense discomfort.

I attended these heat therapy sessions every week and as the temperature intensified over my bare buttocks, I learnt to endure my escalating anguish.

Once again I was sent back to my GP because I wasn't improving and a second CT scan showed nothing had changed. No cause for the pain was identified and no lumbar disc prolapses were seen.

At this point, instead of persevering with the physiotherapist, he decided to send me to an osteopath for another opinion.

After school, I rode my bike to the osteopathy clinic and sat in the waiting room surrounded by anatomical charts of intimidating human skeletons.

The osteopath beckoned me into his treatment room and asked me what was wrong. I pointed to the spot where I was experiencing pain and he asked me to take off everything but my underwear and lie facedown on the treatment table.

After prodding and poking my spine he finally concluded that my vertebrae must be out of alignment. He sounded confident as he produced a shiny device called an 'activator adjusting instrument' and proceeded to adjust me.

I'd never seen an 'activator' before, but quickly discovered they are commonly used by osteopaths and chiropractors to adjust their patients' joints. They are slightly larger than a pen and are designed to release a low-level force into the underlying joint when the trigger mechanism is released.

The osteopath manoeuvred his way around the base of my spine, clicking and thudding into all the typical places he was used to adjusting, but nothing was happening. Since I wasn't responding, he palpated my sacrum (the posterior part of my pelvis) and found the area of maximal discomfort. He dialled up the force of his 'activator adjusting instrument', aimed at the centre of the target on my back and pressed the trigger.

I'd already endured a lot of physical treatments without flinching or making a sound, but this time I wailed like I'd been hit by an axe. He had definitely found the painful spot and was so pleased that he hit me again, and again, and again, in the same area.

I writhed in agony but didn't complain because I trusted my practitioner.

He asked his receptionist to book me in for regular appointments and I obediently returned each week for my 'activation'. The pain felt worse after every session, but I accepted the punishment and kept going back for six months because I knew this was going to make me better eventually.

I was simultaneously trying to study for my final year of high school but the discomfort was getting worse. Every night I'd turn over in my sleep and be brutally woken by the sharp pain.

One day I arrived at the osteopathy clinic and sat down next to the skeletons that had become very familiar over time. But my usual osteopath wasn't there, and a locum welcomed me into the chamber of horrors. I disrobed and lay facedown on the treatment table. He asked me what was wrong, gently pressed on my sacrum and my pain level hit the ceiling once more. He didn't provide therapy that day but instead wrote a letter to my doctor suggesting a bone scan.

I soon found myself sitting at the hospital radiology unit, watching a syringe of radioactive dye getting pumped into my veins. These radioactive isotopes flowed around my body and were tailored to attach to any areas of abnormal bone growth. The radiologist took a look at my sacrum and the area causing pain lit up like a Christmas tree.

The area in question is a static piece of bone, shaped like a triangle at the back of your pelvis. It's unusual to get pain in the middle of your sacrum because there aren't any moving parts to cause problems.

The GP told me he now had a new diagnosis – this looked like a bone tumour, possibly cancer.

Even though I'd been pointing to my sacrum the whole time, he'd requested a CT scan of the wrong anatomical area – twice.

My next appointment was with a paediatric orthopaedic specialist and I found myself in yet another waiting room, this time surrounded by other teenagers with their limbs in plaster.

An MRI revealed the villain of this story – a lump in exactly the same spot I'd been pointing to for the past few years. It had been slowly growing, was now the size of a walnut, and was the likely cause of my ongoing discomfort.

The physiotherapist's heat treatment had been painful because it encouraged blood flow into the tumour, which caused swelling and increased pressure on the surrounding area.

The osteopath's 'activator' had also caused extreme pain because it tapped directly onto the bony growth.

No amount of heat therapy or hitting me with a stick was going to help. I needed surgery.

Thankfully my parents believed in modern medicine and booked me in for the operation, but they also believed a higher power had the potential to heal me. While we waited for my day in theatre, they encouraged me to try God out first.

I come from a Protestant family and we'd been part of Baptist or Presbyterian communities for years. I'd attended church every Sunday for as long as I could remember, and praying every night was just part of my routine. I was told I needed to pray even harder and more frequently if I wanted God to take this tumour away.

I doubled my prayer efforts. Anything to avoid surgery.

Whenever I had a few spare minutes, I'd pray for God to remove the bony lump in my sacrum. I was praying as I biked to school in the morning, and I'd pray myself to sleep in the evening.

I'd been taught that if I loved God and had enough faith, then I'd be able to move mountains, and he would be able to remove tumours.

One day, after an unusually long prayer session, I was absolutely convinced I'd prayed hard enough. It was then that a tingly feeling flowed from the crown of my head, through my body and all the way down to my lower back. A deep sense inside told me that God had healed me during this prayer time.

However, I was suddenly faced with a religious dilemma. How would I know if I was healed or not?

I'd read the Bible story of 'doubting Thomas', one of Jesus's disciples. After Jesus had been nailed to a crucifix and died, Thomas was the one who said he'd only believe Jesus had come back to life if he was able to see and feel the wounds himself. Jesus then turned up next to Thomas with a disappointed look on his face. Thomas was embarrassed that he had ever doubted. I didn't want to disappoint Jesus and I certainly didn't want to be written up as 'doubting Brad' in a future gospel story.

I knew my faith was strong enough for the tumour to go away, so I didn't need proof that a miracle had occurred. But I needed to know it was gone so I could cancel my surgery. Science collided with religion and I was caught in a Schrödinger's cat quandary.

I needed to touch my back to see if I still had pain. But I was worried that if God had removed the tumour and I started doubting him, maybe he'd sneak it back in again.

The moments between praying and checking were stressful. I quietly slid my hand down my sacral surface to the epicentre of my Schrödinger's tumour. My fingers were poised over the lump that both was and wasn't there. I pressed in and suddenly doubled over in agony and disappointment. What was wrong with me? What was I doing wrong?

My own prayer wasn't working, but my parents told me that God worked in mysterious ways. My mother had spoken with our Catholic neighbour across the road and she suggested we attend a special healing service at her local church. When it comes to getting better from a bone tumour, putting aside centuries of conflict between Catholics and Protestants was surely allowed?

Incense filled my nose as we turned up at the Catholic church. The service commenced and I was encouraged to line up at the front. The priest came out dressed in frilly white robes and proceeded to pray loudly and lay his healing hands on injured body parts. He touched people's heads if they suffered from headaches and held hands if they had arthritis in their fingers.

He approached me and asked what was wrong. I remember thinking that if he was so close to God, he should have already been told what my problem was, but I went along with this spiritual process and told him my tumour was in the middle of my bum. For some reason, he didn't place his healing hands on my buttocks, but touched my forehead instead.

I reminded him that I didn't have a headache, but he still didn't touch below my waist.

I stood at the front of the church with my eyes closed and hands reaching up to heaven. I prayed with the priest for God to remove the tumour from the base of my spine. Tingles flew up and down my body and I knew that God must have worked some magic. The priest blessed me and moved on to pray for the next person in the queue while I walked back to take my seat. I sat down on the hard wooden pew beside my mother and nearly threw up from the pain.

The priest's healing hands on my forehead and a theatrical church service might have given me tingles while I was standing in front of everyone, but away from the incense, the crowds, my mum and our well-meaning neighbour, I felt empty and betrayed.

Maybe if I had prayed even harder? Maybe if the priest had touched my bum? Maybe if I'd eaten more leafy green vegetables?

A few days later, I was admitted to hospital for surgery.

The orthopaedic surgeon made an incision over my sacrum, delicately removed the bone tumour from my nerves and sent it off for testing.

The surgeon was happy with my progress and after six days he discharged me. The final pathology result came back with a diagnosis of an osteoblastoma – a very rare, but thankfully benign bone tumour.

My family was thrilled I didn't have cancer. They started praising God for getting me through the operation, but I found their attitude perplexing because God hadn't done anything.

What made me better was the dedication, hard work and nimble hands of my paediatric orthopaedic specialist.

These events were traumatising as a teenager because I had no idea what to expect. Before the operation, I didn't know if I would become a paraplegic, expire on the operating table, or if they would find cancer and I'd succumb to a prolonged, painful and gruesome death.

I was fortunate – my surgeon was skilled. I had no awful side effects from the operation, and many years later I have nothing but a scar to show and a story to share from the experience.

It was a lot for me to get my head around, made all the more stressful because by this time I was trying to finish my final-year high school exams.

I had placed trust in my doctor but was unfortunately misdiagnosed. I had trusted my physiotherapist and osteopath, but they had unknowingly tortured me for months without benefit. I had put my faith in God, but my faith was misplaced.

It taught me a valuable lesson. My experience as a patient helped me understand the embarrassment, vulnerability and anxiety people can feel when they engage with doctors and try to navigate a confusing healthcare system.

I also saw just how easy it was – when faced with an overwhelming diagnosis, a painful treatment or confusing medical advice – to be lured towards alternative therapies that might sound more promising, more optimistic and less painful.

As my final year of school came to a close, I applied to study medicine.

CHAPTER 2

ROOT CAUSE

We expect our bodies to work perfectly, and when they betray us we want to know why.

We often try to identify a direct cause and effect, like 'I drank too much alcohol therefore I threw up', but life isn't always so simple.

The cause of illness can be complex and often the result of many factors. It's our unique combination of genetics, environment and lifestyle choices that increase or decrease the chance we'll get sick. Some deep digging and research into someone's history can often unveil the reasons why they were more likely to develop ill health.

There are some diseases, however, that physicians label as 'idiopathic', which essentially means we have no idea what caused them.

'Idiopathic pulmonary fibrosis' fits into this category. This is the official name of a medical condition where scar tissue accumulates within someone's lungs and breathing becomes increasingly difficult. Doctors can describe the pathological process and we know what the cells look like under a microscope, but we don't know what causes this condition to occur.

The osteoblastoma I was diagnosed with fits into this 'idiopathic' category as well, but as a young man I struggled to accept that there was no reason for its development. What had I done wrong to develop such a rare bone tumour? I was keen to find out when I started medical school.

Excited and curious, I turned up to our lecture on benign bone tumours, ready to take notes. Our professor explained that bone tumours were rare and he planned to run through all the different types over the following sixty minutes. By the end of the hour he hadn't mentioned anything about osteoblastomas. I raised my hand and asked why, and he told me not to worry about them, 'They're so rare, you'll never see one in your lifetime,' and then, without waiting for me to respond, he packed up his gear and left.

It was a bit of a letdown because I didn't discover anything more about the rare tumour that had caused me so much anguish.

What we do know is that osteoblastomas are more likely to occur in children and in males, but we don't know why. Bone tumours grow slowly from a single cell, but it's unclear what makes that initial cell mutate in the first place.

Our bodies contain over 30 trillion cells, so there's a decent chance something can go wrong in one of them.

University taught me that life is a lottery, and we may never know why we're dealt the cards we get. But this jarred with what I'd been taught at church – that everything happens for a reason.

I'd learnt that we all live in a spiritual landscape with angels and demons in constant battle for our souls. Reality was merely our perception and if we drew back the curtain clouding our spiritual vision, we'd glimpse the heavenly realm and understand the true cause behind the plight of humanity.

Religious concepts had been drummed into my head and so I came to the conclusion God had punished me for something I'd done by placing a painful tumour into my back. The most obvious abomination I could think of was that I'd had a crush on a boy at school.

No one knew I was attracted to men, but I was sure God knew.

At primary school in New Zealand, there were telltale signs of my impending sexuality. It might be a bit of a stereotype, but you'd never find me on the field playing rugby – I'd be in the school corridor playing elastics with the girls. Inside was much warmer in winter, you didn't get covered in mud, and I was much better at jumping over stretched hurdles than kicking a football. As I approached puberty, I was more attracted to my own gender than the opposite sex, but I'd been told it wasn't the natural order of the world.

In all my juvenile wisdom, I concluded that the funny feeling I got in my pelvis around certain guys must have directly caused one of my bone cells to mutate into a tumour. After surgery I felt like I'd faced God's wrath and learnt my lesson, so of course now I would be straight.

But being straight didn't come that easy.

Towards the end of my medical degree, I plucked up enough courage to speak with my trusted friend Carolyn about my problem and I explained that being gay was probably the cause of my tumour.

She replied, 'I think you're right, but for the wrong reasons. It's not a punishment from God, you just brought it on yourself. I heard of a woman who was sexually abused and started hating her vagina. After years of disliking her genitals, she ended up giving herself cervical cancer. Maybe it's the same for you, feeling so distressed about your sexuality that you willed the tumour to grow.'

Initially I thought her theory could have merit until I realised the tumour would have developed in my penis if that were the case. I winced at the thought.

I knew deep down that, scientifically, it didn't make sense. My medical education had taught me that people don't give themselves cervical cancer. The vast majority of cervical cancers are caused by the Human Papilloma Virus (HPV), a common infection transmitted during sexual contact. The virus causes cervical cells to grow abnormally and, over years, they sometimes turn cancerous.

There's always an explanation behind someone's suffering in the Bible. They might have done something wrong and God is punishing them. They might have done something right but Satan is testing their faith. There's even the concept of 'generational sin', where someone's ancestor did something wrong and suffering perpetuates throughout their family line forever.

'Generational sin' sounded more like victim blaming to me. Illness passed from one generation to the next is much more likely to be a genetically inherited disease than divine intervention.

Humans knew nothing about genetics when the Bible was written, but now we know that the causes of many diseases are due to the coding in our DNA. In biblical times, people would be thrown out of the city gates for being possessed by demons, but they probably just had epilepsy.

Some things just happen randomly – that's life. We can't explain why they occur, and attempting to ascribe meaning where meaning is not there is a futile process.

But that's what we do. We're human. We look for patterns and associations to explain the world around us. Sometimes we're right, but often we're wrong. Science helps us to acknowledge our fallibility, put aside our personal perception of the world and step into an objective environment. It takes time, it's a difficult process, but it's worthwhile if we want to create a space of humility where we are not just fooling ourselves.

I can understand why people believe celebrities and influencers who offer answers online. When your mother develops Parkinson's disease and you're searching to find the root cause, attributing blame to fluoride, 5G or junk food can be cognitively comforting, even if it's incorrect.

It's often easier to direct anger or hatred towards a radio tower sitting on a hill than accept that sometimes horrible things happen to good people.

We've all heard the phrase 'Everything happens for a reason', but reality is much more messy. Bad people can skate through life without any comeuppance or retribution, while good people can be mercilessly hit with one illness after another. No one is wholly good or bad all the time, so this further complicates the reasoning.

The universe isn't perpetually balanced by good and evil forces, but this theory has persisted for millennia, steeped into the myths, fables and stories we are told as children. Angels and demons, Yin and Yang, Jedis and Sith lords, even karmic forces assume an overriding cosmic control.

This is how we think of other people and even ourselves, a balance sheet of right and wrong. My own experience was to focus only on my sexuality and to accept that my bone tumour was a punishment.

●

Towards the end of my studies I understood that being gay wasn't something I had chosen, wasn't something I could change, and hadn't given me a bone tumour.

But this conflicted with my religious beliefs and my emotional stress was growing. I felt an increasing drive to come out to my friends and family, but I didn't want to disappoint anyone. Coming out would essentially mean losing many of my childhood friends and possibly cause me to be ostracised from my church community.

People struggling with their sexuality can remain closeted for years, living in constant fear of their secret being exposed. They endure ongoing inner turmoil because it's too painful to contemplate an alternative.

Around this time I was experiencing an overwhelming sense of tiredness. It was an effort to get up every morning and I felt a heaviness throughout my entire body. Every day it felt like I was walking through water. I felt unwell all the time. I found it difficult to cope with my hospital rounds as a medical student, and at the end of the day I'd have a quick nap in the car before driving home.

My GP requested some blood tests, but everything looked fine and they reassured me that I'd likely get better soon.

Six months went by and nothing changed. My sleep had been terrible while the osteoblastoma festered at the base of my spine and now it had become fragmented again.

All day I'd feel wrecked but climbing into bed at night triggered a wave of insomnia that refused to let me sleep. Lying in the darkness I would feel shattered but unable to pass out.

When I did fall unconscious, restful slumber evaded me, and I would be plunged into a series of nightmares – compelled to fight for my own survival until daylight.

Opening my eyes in the morning I'd look around the room, but find my body frozen in place. I'd eventually break free from my night-time demons and join the living for another day of heavy eyelids and exhaustion.

As a hospital resident I scheduled regular coffee breaks throughout my day so I could get through a nine-hour shift. I'd drive home, have a nap, and then wake up for dinner before going back to sleep again. My life was literally work and sleep because I didn't have much energy for anything else.

By this time, I'd had multiple blood tests and seen several doctors who were unsure what to tell me. The diagnosis most consistent with my pattern of symptoms was glandular fever followed by a post-viral fatigue syndrome. The majority of people who develop glandular fever bounce back within a couple of weeks, some people take six months to recover, but by this time I'd been struggling for years.

Post-viral fatigue might sound impressive, but this vague diagnosis was less than satisfactory. Treatment options were even less exhilarating: watch and wait and hope things improve.

I wasn't getting answers from doctors so I started wondering whether the constant fear of coming out was draining my energy. Even though the healing prayer service hadn't worked when I was a teenager, the church elders had continued to assure me that God answered prayers. So I went to another prayer meeting, this time at a Pentecostal church in Melbourne.

A bunch of congregation members all sat in a circle of chairs in the church hall. Elders were assigned to each person and they approached to ask us what we required from prayer. I told them I felt tired all the time and didn't know what was wrong with me, and I also thought that I might be gay. The church minister looked visibly concerned, placed his hands on my shoulders and started to pray for the demon of fatigue and the demon of same-sex attraction to be taken from me.

There were about twenty people receiving prayer in the same hall and over a few minutes, the church elders' voices became louder and more animated. The praying, mumbling and speaking in tongues crescendoed and the people receiving prayer were standing, sitting, crying, shouting, falling over and even lying on the ground shaking.

I sat on the chair feeling nothing. I was disappointed but sincerely wanted to be healed. I was sick of feeling tired all the time and I didn't want to have a sexuality that would go against what the church wanted for me. I prayed really hard for God to rid my body of those sleepy gay demons.

The minister commanded the demons to come out of my body, and in that moment with everyone wailing around me, I felt a warm sensation gradually rise up within my chest. I imagined a hot demon squirming around inside me, being banished from my body. The feeling rose up from my chest, into my throat, and I envisioned the spiritual beast exiting my mouth and being gone forever.

By this time, I was standing with my eyes closed and my hands held to the sky. I was thanking God for healing me while the minister placed his hands on my forehead.

When your eyes are closed, it's perfectly normal to rock backwards and forwards a little, in order to maintain your balance. The minister's hands constantly pressed onto my forehead, so when I rocked back, he'd move his hand with me, but when I rocked forward, he'd stop me. The natural cadence of my wavering stance continued and, with every subtle movement, I found myself tilted back a little further. Eventually I was tilted so far back that I fell into the catcher's arms and was laid down on the floor like a spiritual sack of potatoes. The minister hooted in triumph, 'Hallelujah. Praise Jesus!' and immediately moved on to pray for the next person in the circle.

•

Falling over at church is pretty common for Pentecostals. Being 'slain in the spirit' is meant to be a sign that people are so overwhelmed by God, they lose control of their muscles and fall to the ground. Everyone reacts a little differently with many shaking, crying, laughing or just lying stiff as a board.

The minister of the church will usually pray for a minute or two before someone becomes 'slain in the spirit', but if God is in a hurry they'll just tap someone's forehead and get the same effect. Some people are more resistant and the minister yells, hisses and claps their hands until God finally enters the person's body and makes them collapse.

This practice is so common that volunteers at Pentecostal churches are assigned as 'catchers'. Burly, male churchgoers are given the weekly task to stand behind people and catch their fall. The catcher's job is to gently lower them to the ground, making sure they don't hurt themselves – imagine how awful it would be if people fell over, full of God's love, and injured themselves in the process.

Unfortunately this did happen at a Pentecostal church I attended. The minister put out an altar call and invited everyone to come up for prayer. As all the catchers were on their way, a member of the congregation suddenly fell over. This was odd because the minister would usually be within their vicinity as a conduit for God's power, but we were frequently told God works in mysterious ways. We initially thought this member of the church must have been slain in the spirit without any human intervention.

He writhed around on the floor with all of his muscles shaking while church members gathered round, praising the Lord for filling him up with the Holy Spirit. This was all good for the first few minutes, until someone noticed blood dripping from the back of his head. The Lord hadn't slain him. He had epilepsy and unfortunately had suffered a grand mal seizure which made him collapse. He'd hit his head in the process and lacerated the back of his scalp. The church leaders realised and sheepishly called an ambulance.

●

Lying on the ground with my eyes closed, I was quite aware I hadn't been slain. It felt like the minister had expected me to fall over and intensified his prayer and forehead pressure until I eventually did.

The weird and spooky sensation I felt in my chest was unlikely to have come from God. It's common to feel strange things, especially when you're in a highly suggestible environment. Maybe you've been in a 'haunted castle' and felt a cool breeze on the back of your neck and then the hair on your head started to prickle. Or you've listened to an orchestra playing such beautiful music that you started welling up with tears. Perhaps you've heard someone sing a note so pure and magical that it hit the sweet spot and you felt at peace with the world.

Standing in the middle of a prayer room, surrounded by people yelling, singing, chanting and mumbling in tongues is a similar experience. Emotions are triggered and we can easily be influenced to believe we're experiencing something supernatural.

At first I was suspicious that I had just been pushed over by a church elder, but I was optimistic that God had cleansed me of my demons. Confident the prayer had worked, I praised the Lord that I was now healed from debilitating fatigue and no longer suffered from what the church had labelled 'Same-sex Attraction Disorder' (SAD). Lying on the ground I peered around the room and locked eyes with the muscular, hot, handsome Christian catcher who had caught me. Maybe I hadn't got rid of my SAD, but I knew I was exhausted after all that prayer and needed a nap.

●

Formalising a diagnosis is a process of elimination. I had made a list of potential reasons for my fatigue and was crossing them out one by one. I'd excluded organic reasons, persistent infections, and my recent exorcism had also ruled out demon possession.

The next step in this science experiment was to tackle the cause of my anxiety head on. I needed to come out to my family – so I did. It didn't go well.

They refused to believe anyone could be attracted to someone of the same sex and told me it wasn't part of God's plan for my life. They thought I must have been hanging out with the wrong kind of people and been deceitfully recruited into a gay sect, but I'd been working so much that I didn't have enough spare time for such extracurricular activities.

It felt like a heavy weight had been taken off my chest after I came out to my folks. Some of my anxiety had diminished but the fatigue persisted.

As my family tried to make sense of my sexuality, they reached out for support within their Christian community. It was the mid-2000s and they were put in contact with an ex-gay ministry called 'Living Waters Australia'. This group had links to 'Exodus International', an overarching organisation dedicated to straightening out gay people.[1]

My sister met a psychologist at one of their prayer sessions and thought he might be able to help me out. The relationship with my immediate family was fracturing, so I agreed to see him.

●

The chair squeaked as I sat down for my first psychotherapy session in the eastern suburbs of Melbourne. The combined fragrance of black mould and artificial air freshener wafted through the room.

The psychologist was softly spoken and in the first five minutes he told me that he was a Christian and didn't believe homosexuality was part of God's plan. He explained he could work with me provided that I was committed to becoming straight.

This initial meeting rang alarm bells because my professional understanding was that a psychologist was meant to provide a non-judgemental environment where their client felt comfortable to explore their ideas and issues. It's the client's prerogative to set the agenda and come to their own conclusions, but not the psychologist's place to inform the direction of treatment before even making an assessment.

I was also quite sure there was an ethical obligation for psychologists to respect their client's personal beliefs and not to impress their own beliefs onto their patient.

I didn't realise it at the time, but I was essentially subjected to a mild form of conversion therapy – an outdated practice that attempted to make gay men and lesbian women straight. The general principle explained to me at the time was that I was broken and needed to ask God into my life to fix me.

More barbaric versions of conversion therapy involved forcing people to watch same-sex pornography while administering medication to make them vomit or electrocuting their genitals. I'm kind of lucky that my conversion therapy simply involved chatting in a slightly musty environment.

There's no evidence conversion therapy works and it can be incredibly harmful. It's based on religious principles that I will simply paraphrase as, 'God said being gay is wrong, so it can't be right – now drop your strides and attach these electrodes to your willy.'

Same-sex attraction was thought to be behaviour that was learnt over time and therefore could be reprogrammed – but this is not the case.

We understand now that same-sex attraction is a normal variation of human behaviour.[2]

In 1973 the American Psychiatric Association concluded that homosexuality wasn't a mental health diagnosis and removed it from the *Diagnostic and Statistical Manual of Mental Disorders*. However, conversion therapy continues today and is well known to cause lasting psychological injuries as people try to force their gay brain to think heteronormative thoughts.[3]

I attended regular psychotherapy sessions but didn't feel more straight and didn't notice any improvement in my fatigue – so I crossed off 'being a closeted gay' from my list of possible reasons for feeling tired.

Thankfully the dangerous and harmful practice of conversion therapy has been outlawed in many Australian states and territories, but unfortunately many people still hold these archaic and dangerous beliefs.

Fatigue is one of the symptoms of depression, so this was the next diagnosis on my list. I decided to make some changes to my life – I put my general practice training on hiatus and went travelling overseas.

Like many other Australians I backpacked around South America, hopping from hostel to hostel and realised I didn't have a care in the world. I wasn't depressed and yet still found it difficult getting up in the morning.

My fellow travellers would wake up early to explore the area in which we were staying but I'd still be sleeping in well after they had gone. I'd eventually awake but even then I'd need to have numerous coffees before hitting the bustling streets.

When I returned home, I was still feeling tired. I felt more comfortable in my own skin, wasn't depressed and with time had accepted that my sacral tumour was just one of the random things that happens in someone's life.

It's difficult to fix your health problems if you don't know what's causing them. I realised my frustration with a lack of someone or something to blame for my woes had left my mind free to fill the gaps with outlandish hypotheses. We often revert to primitive thought patterns of mysticism, spirits, demons or other narratives in order to ascribe blame.

Struggling for energy each day, I chose to move to Coffs Harbour for a sea change. It would be years before I finally discovered the cause of my fatigue, but without a diagnosis I was keen to see if the fresh sea air would do me some good.

CHAPTER 3

DR GOOGLE

When I was a teenager, I received bad health advice from my local community – family, friends, churchgoers and even health professionals. These days I can receive similarly bad information anywhere I go from the convenience of my pocket. Google, Facebook, and even my Instagram feed have the potential to be a constant stream of convenient, but incorrect guidance.

Social media has changed our lives forever. The way human beings interact will never be the same again – but there are both positives and negatives that come from communicating online.

On the positive side we're now able to share information more quickly and freely than ever before. On the negative side we're now able to share misinformation more quickly and freely than ever before.

Scrolling through Facebook it's common to see the same health-related memes pop up in your feed over and over again. Every now and then I see a meme that makes me actually lol.

As in actually laugh out loud, not just exhale through my nose and smile to myself.

My favourite of these is the one that says 'Put onions in your socks while you sleep to fight off a cold or flu', or some variant thereof. In our pre-scientific days raw onion was portrayed as the secret behind detoxifying your body and purifying your blood. Chemicals were thought to be absorbed through the skin on the soles of your feet and float through your body along meridian energy highways to all of your major organs. This process was based on principles of reflexology, where your foot is said to be inextricably linked to your vital organs. However, there are no special onion-absorbing channels in your skin, meridian lines are fictitious with no anatomical basis and there is no scientific reason to explain why onion juice would purify your blood.

A family member recently posted a similar version on her Facebook page recommending friends place a poultice of raw onions on their chest while they sleep at night to help heal a chest infection.

At best, the tart whiff of an onion might be able to penetrate into the swollen tissue of your blocked nose, but your skin acts as a barrier, protecting you from the outside world and any potential detoxifying juices will not be absorbed through your chest wall and into your lungs. It certainly doesn't absorb a raw onion poultice. If your skin were that porous, you'd be able to absorb all the nutrients from your evening meal by smearing spaghetti bolognese over your chest.

The other suggested mechanism of action is to say the onion draws out the infection by sucking out all the bacteria and excess fluid contained in your lungs, but this doesn't happen either.

Whenever these kind of posts appear on my feed I invariably wonder why anybody would ever think this would work – then I'll usually post a chirpy comment underneath, kindly reprimanding my friend or family member for being so gullible.

It is a fact that storing a raw onion in your socks overnight will make your feet reek of onion, but it will not improve your health. However, enough people must believe it's true because this rumour continues to circulate.

During the sixteenth century, diseases were thought to be transmitted through the air within noxious gases and putrid smells. The aroma from chopped onions was therefore believed to offer protection for household members, and families would diligently prepare bowls of this rancid potpourri to distribute throughout their home.

Looking back, we now know this was a waste of time. Bacteria, viruses, parasites, protozoa and prions spread infection, even when you and your loved ones are surrounded by onions.

However, even though we know the onion stench wouldn't have directly protected families from the plague, it is likely that it would have caused a collateral benefit. Physical distancing works during a pandemic and a house full of diced raw onions would have discouraged many potentially infected visitors.

But pandemics are complicated, and transmission of infection would have been impacted by many factors. Households that were able to fund a steady supply of onions would have been more financially secure than those who couldn't afford copious amounts of the root vegetable. In turn, wealthier families would have been able to run a more hygienic home and it could have been judicious cleaning and more frequent bathing that further decreased the chance of transmission. However, it seems like onions were inappropriately bestowed with all the credit.

I've seen onion advocates suggest that consuming onions is a great way to enhance your immune system because some of the chemicals contained within have antibacterial and antiviral qualities. This claim is regularly applied to many foods and supplements but it's misleading because these qualities are generally only found in a research laboratory setting. Eating onions as part of your evening meal is very different from drizzling onion juice over bacteria sitting in a petri dish, which is different again from shoving them in your socks.

It's incredible to think that health rumours like this have persisted as part of human folklore for centuries and have been reinvented as modern social media clickbait.

It's not just onions – there are plenty of other myths that keep finding new life.

Rubbing a gold wedding band on your eyelid will not get rid of a stye – even if the soluble form of gold does have some anti-inflammatory properties. A select number of patients with arthritis may be treated with gold injections or tablets, but generally we have more effective medications with fewer side effects. The gold contained in your grandmother's wedding ring is inert and will not be absorbed through your skin.

Some people swear the gold ring treatment works because they have seen it with their own styes, but eye infections come and go by themselves over time. If you've ever rubbed a gold ring on your stye and noticed it gone the next day, it would have disappeared anyway.

Unfortunately Google searches often don't provide clear and concise information to properly counter these ideas.

Dr Google is in everyone's pocket, always available, never takes a holiday. It dishes out health advice and never asks for money or a Medicare card in return. It's clearly everybody's favourite physician and many of my patients have already consulted with this trusted companion before entering my clinic.

In fact, according to the head of Google Health, David Feinberg, about seven per cent of all Google searches are health-related – that's 70,000 medical queries every minute.[1]

Even though it appears confident with its diagnosis, Dr Google is not always correct. A 2020 study done by Edith Cowan University in Western Australia found that symptom checking websites and apps gave correct advice only about a third of the time.[2] If a trained health professional got diagnoses wrong so often there would be some serious questions asked by the medical board.

Lupus, cancer and rare genetic diseases are often suggested and then it's up to medical doctors like myself to perform a proper assessment, provide a correct diagnosis and deliver counselling to alleviate the undue anxiety caused by the search engine doctor.

Often during a routine consultation I'll provide a diagnosis and my patient will inform me, 'That's what I read online, but I wanted to get your opinion to see if it was right.'

Some of my colleagues see Dr Google as their arch nemesis and advise their patients never to search symptoms, but positives can still be gleaned from the process. I regularly speak with my patients about what the search engine has told them. This line of questioning not only opens up a conversation but gives me an insight into their worst fears. The purpose of a medical consultation often isn't just to get the right diagnosis, it's also to calm our patient's worries, and it can be easier to talk about them with your real doctor if a heartless computer has mentioned them first.

Yet some patients unfortunately remain convinced that their Google search is more trustworthy than seeing a real human doctor.

More than ever before, many people in Australia have easy access to healthy food, premium health services and the latest scientific research, but we've never been more suspicious of healthcare providers.

Social media platforms happily profit from clicks, without any real care whether the online content clicked is helpful or harmful.

So who can you trust?

When I was brought into the world, my family lived by a little stream in the Hutt Valley near Wellington. Our family GP had deep-set eyes, spoke with a reverberating voice like Kamahl and smelled of cigarettes.

Back in those good old days, most people placed their trust in the local family doctor. We believed what our doctor told us, and generally their diagnosis was correct. But, of course, there weren't many other options available.

In our family home the only resource was a medical encyclopedia. Occasionally we would thumb through the pages attempting to match our symptoms with a condition in the book. We couldn't google any weird rashes so we needed to block our noses to brave our GP's tobacco-scented breath and emerge from his clinic with whatever knowledge he decided to bestow upon us.

The internet wasn't available until after I'd started university. Students needed to hang out at the library and navigate through the Dewey Decimal System to find an appropriate textbook. Sometimes we'd resort to microfiche and spend endless hours scrolling through catalogued information until our academic curiosity had been appropriately satisfied.

Access to online information is now an intuitive part of our lives, but in the early days of the internet we had special tutorials at university designed to teach the class how to use this brand new search engine called 'Google'. We gained so much space in our homes because we no longer needed to store copious volumes of *Encyclopedia Britannica* along the length of our bedrooms.

This access to information is wonderful and powerful and gives patients more autonomy over their own health. We should never go back to the days when knowledge about health was held only by those with a medical degree.

But interpreting what's accurate and credible takes practice. It's difficult to tease out facts from fiction, especially when facts are jumbled up with rumours, myths or barefaced lies.

Some time spent researching online – or sharing a pretty meme on your social media feed – does not arm people with enough information when it comes to complicated and important issues like health care. Taking everything with a grain of salt is key. You can't believe everything you read, and a healthy dose of scepticism might be the answer.

CHAPTER 4

THE WHOLE PANTRY OF LIES

We're suckers for a classic fairy tale. We love to cheer on the underdog and clap for the beautiful maiden when she perseveres against all odds to rise triumphantly from the ashes.

Belle Gibson's life story was one of those fairy tales we desperately wanted to believe was true. She fought the dark forces of brain cancer with organic food and a few cheeky coffee enemas, but instead of rising like a phoenix from the ashes, this beautiful maiden turned into the villain of her own story.

Belle's fairy tale began in 2009 when she was in her late teens – the prime of your life, when you feel like anything is possible. But Belle received some terrible news. She was diagnosed with metastatic cancer, with tumours identified in her brain, liver, kidneys, spleen and uterus. Her prognosis obviously wasn't great and she was given four months to live.

When you're diagnosed with cancer, it's a race against time. Medical staff are keen to act quickly to either stop the cancer before it has time to spread further, or to give you the best quality of life for the time you have left.

Belle did what most people would do when they are diagnosed with cancer. She diligently followed her doctor's advice and attended the oncology unit to commence chemotherapy and radiotherapy sessions.

●

Hospitals can be scary places full of serious expressions, solemn mumbles and disorientating corridors. Thin polyester curtains rustle between beds, wards are brightly illuminated by flickering fluorescent lights and plastic hoses extend from the walls like cyberpunk octopuses.

Removing your clothing, plucking out piercings and placing your personal possessions onto a plastic tray makes you feel stripped of your identity. Stepping into a flimsy pair of disposable underwear and attempting to cover yourself with an open-backed surgical gown is undignified and only made worse by the accumulation of sweat, tears and bloodstains as you're poked, prodded and punctured by medical procedures.

Modern cancer treatments include surgery, chemotherapy and radiotherapy. They are generally unpleasant, involve plenty of time away from home and come with side effects – so it's not uncommon for people to seek alternative cancer treatments that are less intense. Unfortunately less intense cancer treatments are frequently fatal.

Belle Gibson pursued medical treatment for a couple of months on the oncology ward, but eventually found it was too much to handle. Risking everything, she swapped modern medicine for what she saw to be a more holistic approach and embarked on a quest to treat her cancer naturally by educating herself online.

She researched alternative cancer therapies and created her own combined treatment regimen of superfoods, vitamins and natural medicine. She embraced a vegetarian diet, which included organic food and excluded gluten and sugar. She practised meditation and relaxation strategies, underwent oxygen therapy (breathing high concentrations of oxygen) and regularly evacuated her bowel with enemas made of coffee.

Belle found her own natural treatment regimen seemed to be working well. She was not only surviving cancer but thriving. She had proven her doctors wrong and her story provided inspiration and hope for others surviving cancer across Australia and throughout the world.

She shared her journey over Instagram and rapidly became insta-famous for beating brain cancer through healthy eating. She motivated thousands of people to optimise their own health by following her simple daily routine, and she eventually leveraged this popularity to launch her very own wellness app, The Whole Pantry, in 2013 – four years after her diagnosis.

The Whole Pantry app enabled Belle to share recipes, lifestyle advice and her success story with the world. Supported by Apple, it was downloaded more than two hundred thousand times in the first month of release. Her story was profiled in *The Australian Women's Weekly, Cosmopolitan, Mamamia, marie claire* and *Elle* magazine. The team at *Elle* were so impressed with her story that they named her the 'most inspiring woman you've met this year' in their December 2014 edition.[1]

She negotiated a book deal with Penguin Random House and The Whole Pantry was to be launched as one of the preferred apps on Apple's brand new smart watch.[2]

It was a triumph that she had lived for so many years after having been told she only had a few months to live. How did she do it? Had the doctors been wrong? Was the secret to beating cancer just a healthy diet all along? Would other patients be able to keep their cancer at bay by following her advice too? Why use chemotherapy and radiotherapy if all you need to do is eat cleanly?

Belle modelled herself as a shining example of someone who had it all worked out. Defeating cancer was as easy as eating The Whole Pantry, and if she could do it, you could too. Her app didn't just contain recipes, she was selling hope.

I wish the fairy tale ended here, where Belle Gibson and her followers discover the cure for cancer is organic food and coffee enemas, and everyone lives happily ever after. But the cure for cancer doesn't come from caffeinating your bottom.

Belle's story was far from over and the first fact we need to disclose in order to unpick this fairy tale is that Belle Gibson never had cancer.

●

As a GP, I get to know my patients and their families very well. You watch as people get married, you diagnose pregnancies, and then get to see those pregnancies grow up into little people. It's a privilege to see teenagers bumble their way through asthma, acne, broken arms, broken hearts and finally find their way to adulthood. It also tears your heart apart when some of those young patients develop brain cancer.

Symptoms can be as subtle as forgetting people's names or as spectacular as having a seizure.

Unfortunately the treatments available aren't great.

If you have brain cancer, a neurosurgeon needs to open your cranium and remove as much of it as possible while trying to leave your normal brain tissue intact. The tumour is cut into slices and examined under a microscope so the pathologist can make a determination about how aggressive it is, how far it may have spread and whether they think they got it all out.

Brain surgery leaves you with a shaved head and a scar, and hopefully without a stroke.

It's followed by chemotherapy – where your veins are filled with chemicals intent on killing the cells betraying your body; or radiotherapy – where your skull is strapped into a vice while your head is targeted with a beam of radiation; or both.

For some people the treatment is very successful. For others, pursuing active treatment might give them an extra year at best, but most of that time could be spent in hospital.

Any medical treatment is a balance of pros and cons. There is no one-size-fits-all answer when it comes to quantity versus quality of life, and part of the artistry of oncology is to offer tailored treatments to suit each individual patient.

But this didn't have to be your life if you followed Belle Gibson's holistic advice. Doing things her way, you were given the chance to avoid all that horrible nastiness. No operations, radiotherapy, chemotherapy or side effects. Just tasty meals, a regenerated brain and a long life like hers.

Despite her cancer diagnosis, Belle Gibson was a picture of health and a vast community of supportive followers were drawn to her incredible story. She sold false hope to vulnerable people, served on a magnificent plate of kale.

•

There were issues with her story from the beginning. She claimed her health problems commenced after receiving an immunisation against cervical cancer. She blamed the vaccine for giving her a stroke and then blamed the stroke for turning into brain cancer. A significant claim, which, like so much of Belle Gibson's story, would prove false.

The HPV vaccine started being given to young women in Australia from 2007, and while it protects people from developing cancer related to the wart virus, it is not known to cause strokes.

Strokes are either ischaemic (a blockage of blood supply to part of the brain) or haemorrhagic (a bleed into brain tissue). Brain cancer could potentially cause a stroke by blocking or damaging blood vessels in the brain, but a stroke isn't going to cause brain cancer.

Health professionals familiar with her story thought it was improbable but this wasn't as obvious to the general public, who are often wired for optimism. Journalists are meant to be curious and sceptical, but they lapped it up – as did publishers, business executives and especially her fans.

Dr Stephanie Alice Baker is a sociologist from City, University of London. She's the co-author of *Lifestyle Gurus* and has been closely following Belle Gibson and the influencer phenomenon for a long time. She's interested in the way we communicate online, how we interact with each other and how people achieve celebrity and influence in the first place.

Belle Gibson became front-page news in March 2015 when her miraculous story started to unravel. Stephanie recalls that back then 'Instagram was very much in its infancy. So even when she had two hundred thousand followers, that doesn't sound huge now, but it was then.'

At that time, Belle was earning a significant income from selling her success story and through The Whole Pantry app. Belle promised to donate some of her profit to charity organisations, however an investigation by Beau Donelly and Nick Toscano from *The Age* and *The Sydney Morning Herald* revealed these promised donations never showed up. None of the charities had any record of receiving money from Belle Gibson, and four of the five charities didn't even realise fundraising had been organised in their names.[3]

People started asking more questions. Belle defiantly posted a statement on social media reiterating her story – she had given up on conventional treatment and chosen to treat herself naturally. She claimed conventional treatment had made her cancer worse and she was now helping other people fight cancer by using natural therapies.[4]

Her incredible tale continued to crumble and in April 2015, Belle Gibson admitted in an interview with *The Australian Women's Weekly* that she had never actually been diagnosed with cancer by a medical doctor and that no part of her story was true.[5]

She had remained a picture of health because she wasn't dying from cancer. She had never had cancer.

Consumer Affairs Victoria took her case to the Federal Court and in 2017 she was found guilty of misleading and deceptive conduct and fined $410,000.[6] She failed to pay any of the fine and in January 2020 her home was raided by Victoria's Sheriff's Office in an attempt to recoup funds.[7]

The Whole Pantry app was pulled by Apple and her book publisher, Penguin, made a donation of $30,000 to the Victorian Consumer Law Fund. Consumer Affairs Victoria recommended that Penguin must 'enhance its compliance, education and training program with a specific focus on ensuring all claims about medical conditions are substantiated, and that statements about natural therapies are accompanied by a prominent warning notice'.[8]

●

It's difficult to know just how many people were negatively influenced by Belle Gibson's actions. We don't know how many cancer sufferers followed her advice and were devastated when they were unable to recreate her success. It's possible that very sick people delayed treatment to follow her futile regimen.

Dr Stephanie Alice Baker gave me more of an insight into how broad Belle's fanbase was at the time. 'It wasn't just cancer patients,' she said. 'It's very easy to point the finger at them and say, "Oh, it was just people in search of a miracle cure," but it wasn't.

'The people who were invested in her narrative were people like you and me who might have an interest in health, they might be academics, they might be practitioners. A lot of people were duped, and that certainly wasn't limited to people who directly experienced cancer or knew somebody, like a loved one, who had cancer,' Stephanie explained.

Belle went to great lengths to fabricate her narrative and mislead more than two hundred thousand followers. It's a fantastical story that seems impossible with hindsight, so why did so many people fall for it?

Associate Professor Darren Saunders is a cancer researcher who closely followed Belle Gibson's journey because of his own interest in cancer cures – real ones.

I asked Darren why Belle Gibson was so effective at engaging with her audience and he reflected that online influencers are 'very, very good at connecting with their audience, offering simple solutions to often complex problems. They are also very skilful in their ability to understand the fears and anxieties of their audience, and how to connect to those fears and anxieties.'

Darren explained that 'people want to buy into the image and lifestyle that influencers project or represent'.

Online influencers are true to their name – they are influential – but their charismatic power and ability to engage with their audience can be used for honest or nefarious purposes. In an effort to understand why influencers would ignore science or reject medical advice about something as serious as cancer, Darren suggests, 'No doubt some are genuinely trying to help, even if misguided. Others are suffering narcissistic delusions about their own ability or insight, and others are clearly very cynically engaging in marketing and sales exercises. Some are a mix of all three.'

One of the more outrageous parts of Belle Gibson's tale is just how influential she became without anyone thoroughly checking her credentials. Who was responsible for fact-checking Belle's story?

Stephanie commented that in this situation, 'a lot of people didn't do their checks.'

But asking someone to prove they have brain cancer seems like such an odd request – even rude. It could be interpreted as offensive or disrespectful by someone who is actually incredibly ill. Stephanie told me this may well be true, 'But when you're selling a book and have, in fact, rejected modern medicine, it is in that case a reasonable request.

'There's a responsibility on behalf of the publisher to check credentials,' Stephanie said, 'that's their responsibility because they are publishing it.'

However, she is optimistic that this kind of situation is unlikely to happen again. 'If someone were to have a similar narrative that they put forward, it would be checked. I don't think it will be as easy to dupe people.'

This is an idea shared by Darren who spoke with news.com.au at the time and warned, 'We need to be sceptical of the mythical lone genius selling magical cures that ignore basic science and hard evidence ... Hopefully this will make people think twice and do some basic checking of facts.'[9]

Being diagnosed with a serious health issue can be really tough and when it happens, it's important to have plenty of support from family, friends and trusted health professionals.

Medical teams need to offer treatments based on the latest scientific evidence and therapies proven to work. Procedures and medication may be unpleasant, painful or even expensive, which is why the benefits, risks and potential side effects need to be clearly explained.

It's easy for patients to feel overwhelmed. It's tempting to let any tense moment, tearful argument or unpleasant procedure put them off medical treatment altogether, so it's essential for patients to be engaged and invested in their own health care.

Belle Gibson gave her audience the impression that she was able to leave modern medicine behind and forge a new path for herself. She offered an alternative pathway free from doctors and hospitals. Her false claims could have easily inspired others to follow her example – a decision that could be disastrous.

Health professionals are on your side. It's our job to be realistic and tell you the honest truth, and unfortunately that isn't always pleasant to hear.

The truth may sometimes be uncomfortable, but the alternative can be dangerous.

CHAPTER 5

THE POWER OF INFLUENCERS

Online influencers can feel like friends to us. They're relatable, engaging, charming, have dazzling smiles, bubbly personalities, share witty jokes, and are always waiting to tell us about their day. Sitting in our pockets like real-life Tamagotchis, we feed them with likes, follows and compliments, and along the way we forget that they are primarily salespeople. We watch their carefully curated lives and follow their nifty tips, while they try to sell us shiny products that would surely make our lives better if only we had them in our possession.

Salespeople have existed throughout history, but they've never been able to reach such huge audiences from the comfort of their own homes before.

Unfortunately, the friend in our pocket can also exhibit an inflated sense of self-belief, speak with authority on topics where they have none, and occasionally possess the power and influence to seriously harm us by presenting ill-informed advice.

Charisma is currency – it's always been the key to influencing people. Some of us are gifted with the ability to change minds, influence elections and sell products. But these gifts can be used for good or for bad – influencers who promote 'wellness' can dramatically improve the health of their followers, or they can cause devastating harm. As noted in Associate Professor Saunders' remarks in the previous chapter, the reasons they commence and continue to promote their path to 'wellness' are various, and by no means necessarily stem from any intentional malice. There are so many people working in this space who truly believe in their own health advice.

Enter Sarah Stevenson, stage right.

Sarah has all the aforementioned hallmarks of a social media influencer. She has the perfect teeth, the great hair, and she lives in an Instagrammable house, with the confidence to sit in front of a camera for hours every day, drawing people into her world.

She is one of Australia's most prominent wellness gurus and shares her lifestyle tips and healthy recipes to an audience of nearly 1.5 million subscribers on YouTube, and over 1 million followers on Instagram. Her brand, Sarah's Day, is instantly recognisable to plenty of Australian millennials and zoomers.

She sells a range of skincare products, eyewear, activewear, exercise program ebooks, a timing app for fitness training, an 'inner-health and beauty powder' and some cookie dough–flavoured protein powder.

She's one of a growing group that many refer to as 'wellness warriors'. These are people who sell a healthy, happy lifestyle to their followers, and are able to make money from their masses of online 'friends'.

She always looks fit, energised, refreshed and ready to take on the world – but her photos are notable for prominent product placement.

●

Achieving the state of *wellness* promoted by people like Sarah is not only about living in the absence of disease or illness, but also has the added pressure of needing to maximise your fitness, productivity and enjoyment of life.

In other words, *wellness* is an ethereal concept that is unattainable in the real world. You might feel well on occasion, but you can never reach a state of wellness because there is always something else that you can improve.

We may all strive to achieve this state of being, but everyone is just muddling their way through the world the best way we know how. We can only try to make good decisions for our health, based on our best understanding of the information that's presented to us.

The reality, however, is that *wellness* is an endless pursuit for the privileged – an expensive hobby for those who are already well. The trick of skilful social media influencers is that they make people think they don't have enough, are not healthy enough, or will just find that extra bit of happiness around the next corner.

I'd never heard of the self-proclaimed Holistic Health Princess until I received an email in early 2018 from the pop-culture podcast *Shameless* asking for my opinion about Sarah's latest Instagram post.

Accompanying a very carefree-looking photo of her frolicking on the beach was an enthusiastic missive to her followers, excitedly announcing that she had reversed her cervical dysplasia.

The cogs in my medically trained brain suddenly ground to a halt. Sarah may as well have claimed she made the sun come up this morning.

The cervix is the gateway to the uterus, positioned at the top of the vagina. Unfortunately abnormal cells can develop in the cervix and after many years can eventually turn into cancer. Cervical dysplasia is the medical term used to describe these cells that have mutated but haven't yet become cancerous.

There are different Cervical Intraepithelial Neoplasia (CIN) grades used to describe the severity of the condition. CIN1 means there are only subtle changes, CIN2 means the changes are more obvious and CIN3 is heading towards cervical cancer.

Soon after her excited Instagram announcement Sarah posted a follow up YouTube video, titled 'How I Healed Myself Naturally: Cervical Dysplasia CIN 3 (High Grade)'. The clip starts with Sarah giving the following disclaimer:

> I'm like really excited to film this video, but at the same time I'm really nervous because everything in the health world – especially if it is like a serious health issue, there's just so much backlash and judgement that comes with it, but I'm really trying to like not think about that, and think about you guys and the girls who are watching this video who are currently going through this because

> when I found out that I had cervical dysplasia all I was doing was just like researching every single night so I'm making this video for my past self.[1]

It's quite clear from these opening remarks that her reason for recording this video is to help others who find themselves in the same position.

To summarise the vlog, Sarah had consulted with her gynaecologist who advised her to have surgical treatment for these high grade (CIN3) changes.

Instead of following her doctor's advice she decided to heal her cervix herself after doing 'research' online, praying and creating her own cervical dysplasia diet. Several months after making this lifestyle change, she went back to her gynaecologist to find her cervical dysplasia had improved.

Impressed by her own perceived ability to improve her cervical health, she was now sharing the information with her followers so they knew how to do it too.

Don't get me wrong, promoting a healthy lifestyle is admirable, but believing that you can cure cervical dysplasia by following a particular diet is not grounded in reality as it is not supported by science. When more than a million people follow you online, and young women look up to you as a role model, telling them to diverge from medical advice is, in my view, extremely irresponsible.

The vast majority of cervical cancers are caused by the Human Papilloma Virus (HPV), also known as the virus that causes warts. HPV is very common and most people who have had sex will have HPV somewhere on their body.

HPV often causes cells to grow abnormally on the cervix, but it's common for the human immune system to correct these cells over time without assistance.

The immune system is a marvellous thing, and it's in a constant battle to keep HPV under control. This battle waxes and wanes over the years, leading to periods of time when everything looks normal, followed by periods of time when everything looks much worse.

It's a very complex competition, and you really don't have much control over it. It would be naive to believe that your positive thoughts and consumption of green smoothies are playing a role.

While Sarah may seem convinced in her YouTube video that she was able to take control of the situation in a 'healthy and holistic, natural way', scientific research has never proven a correlation between dietary changes and a reduction in cervical abnormalities. Her advice would be ineffective at the very best, and at the very worst it would be potentially harmful to her fans.

The fact is that Sarah was lucky. Her cervical dysplasia reduced from CIN3 to a lower grade, but this would have happened without investing time in prayer, positive thoughts or special smoothies.

Others following her advice may not be so lucky. In fact, engaging in fanciful practices can delay timely gynaecological interventions and potentially lead to someone developing cervical cancer.

The video is also insulting to people who have been diagnosed with cervical dysplasia and had appropriate treatment, and those who have had cervical cancer. Her 'cervical dysplasia diet' and lifestyle regimen implies that surgical intervention is only required if you haven't prayed hard enough, haven't thought positively enough and haven't consumed the right combination of nutrients.

As I discovered with my bone tumour, sometimes bad things happen and it's unhelpful to play the blame game.

Thankfully we have a fantastic cervical screening program in Australia and most cases of cervical cancer can be avoided by treating abnormal cells before they have the chance to become cancerous. The HPV vaccination (developed in Australia) has also been extremely successful at preventing HPV infection and stopping cancer from developing in the first place.

The 'backlash and judgement' Sarah refers to in the disclaimer at the start of her YouTube video is presumably in response to comments she received about her original Instagram post.

After Michelle Andrews and Zara McDonald refuted the post on their popular *Shameless* podcast, the CEO of Cancer Council Australia, Professor Sanchia Aranda, was swift with her rebuke, saying there is 'no evidence that there is anything a woman can do in terms of diet and lifestyle that promotes regression'.[2]

In the YouTube video Sarah did take time to remind her audience that she was not a medical professional herself:

> ... all I'm doing is sitting here and telling you my story and what I did. Take from that what you will, but especially with your serious health issues I highly recommend and

highly advise you and encourage you to go to your medical professional like your gynaecologist and your doctors or whoever you want to go to and listen to their advice ... and healing myself was actually under the guidance of my gynaecologist and my naturopath, so I was always under medical supervision I guess, but you guys know my love, my passion in life is just healthy eating and I really believe that food is thy medicine, and honestly if you have cervical dysplasia and you've already booked in to get surgery I don't want you to watch this video and think that you're doing something wrong, or you should be doing what I did. There is no right and wrong way to really do anything with your body, it's totally up to you and what you feel confident with and comfortable with. So with that disclaimer done honestly if you're watching this video right now and you're already wanting to rip me to shreds for, like, talking about healthy alternatives you should probably just click off now because the rest of this video is just telling you all of the healthy ways that I cured my cervix.[3]

I asked Dr Stephanie Alice Baker why these disclaimers are used by influencers like Sarah, and she explained that they often believe it gives them permission to talk about anything, 'it absolves influencers of responsibility and the potential for any associated legal consequences'.

This statement is Sarah's version of a 'get out of jail free' card. Influencers like her appear to believe that any consequences from making a health claim – no matter how medically incorrect – are able to be sidestepped by using a similar disclaimer.

It is quite frankly ridiculous for Sarah to say that she is not attempting to provide health advice to her followers by publishing this video.

Stephanie highlighted how 'influencers claim to provide opinions rather than fact', and there's generally no problem when they are discussing the latest fashion trend or smartphone, but the boundary between opinion and advice can become blurry when health topics enter the conversation.

Whether it's intentional or not, Sarah Stevenson follows a pattern that is similar to other online influencers. She's forthcoming, confessional and empathetic to those going through similar experiences and establishes trust with her audience. She's bright, fun, likeable and the more you watch her, the more she feels like a friend. As a result, you're more likely to buy her products without even registering that her online presence is integrated into the company's marketing strategy.

Successful online influencers are able to monetise their opinions and personal lives into a healthy income. They are able to do this whether or not they believe in what they are promoting.

Stephanie is clear about the intention of wellness warriors, stating in her book *Lifestyle Gurus* 'the lifestyles presented online are designed to be inspiring, but they also serve as evidence of the possibilities of self-transformation – who you too could be – if you were to adhere to their lifestyle advice, purchase their books, products or services ... their advice is intended to be facilitative'.[4]

And facilitative it is.

Sarah Stevenson's cervical dysplasia video has been viewed over 360,000 times and has more than 1500 comments. Despite her disclaimer, many comments are from Sarah's fans, thanking her for sharing her knowledge about beating cervical dysplasia.

It's worrying to see so many young people saying that after watching the video they now feel they can overcome their own cervical dysplasia through lifestyle changes. Some even commented that their gynaecologist had recommended urgent surgery but they were instead going to heal themselves using Sarah's advice.

These followers might be gaining some comfort from hearing about Sarah's day, but I can only hope that, alongside the unqualified opinions outlined in her video blog, these impressionable young people are considering the qualified advice from trained health professionals too.

While Sarah Stevenson's advice for healing cervical dysplasia may be worrisome, it's not the only health claim made on her social media platforms.

Her accounts are full of misinformation and pseudoscience, like an immune boosting juice she created to help get rid of a cold. The recipe contains lemon, turmeric powder, black pepper, water, 'gubinge powder' (Kakadu plum) from a brand called Loving Earth, and 'camu camu powder' (Peruvian sour berry) from a brand called Tropeaka. Although this concoction might taste delicious, none of these products is proven to help your body fight off a cold.

In addition to this, and what may not be immediately evident from the recipe and social media post, is that Loving

Earth and Tropeaka have sponsored Sarah's videos in the past. In fact, she has her own range of health powders and nut mixes with these brands. Many of her hardcore fans are already aware of these affiliations as she advertises the products on her website and offers a discount in the comments section below her videos – but it doesn't go unnoticed that the remedy for supposedly beating cervical dysplasia conveniently includes the products she is selling.

This is common throughout Sarah's work. Both brands were mentioned in her cervical dysplasia video, but without any declaration of the commercial relationship.

The desire to be fit and healthy is nothing new. Pick up any women's magazine from the 1950s and you'll see fad diets were commonly featured. False information about health, nutrition and exercise has continued to be spread through the media, but the difference now is the rise of social media stars purporting to be experts in health and nutrition, but devoid of qualifications. And we have much easier access to this poor health advice.

According to the 'Digital 2020: Australia' report, 18 million of us (seventy-one per cent) use social media. Ninety-three per cent of us have a smartphone, and we spend on average five hours and forty-one minutes on the internet per day, one hour and forty-four minutes of which is on social media. Of internet users, ninety-six per cent say they have used a social network or messaging service in the past month.[5]

This provides plenty of opportunity for people like Sarah to spread their message. Social media platforms are constructed to show us things we want to see, reward our brains with dopamine hits, and allow us to curate our own personal feed, full of the beautiful things we find appealing – including the influencer themselves. The algorithms are set up like a gingerbread house in the woods, waiting to attract Hansel and Gretel millennials and zoomers. We're tantalised by the scent of sweet candy, but instead of being fattened up with sugary treats, our bank balance is whittled away.

Cardiothoracic surgeon Dr Nikki Stamp puts it well in her book *Pretty Unhealthy*, 'we live in a world where anti-intellectualism is at an all-time high and people distrust science but will put blind faith in a beautiful person with a smartphone and photo editing software.'[6]

Sarah Stevenson is far from the only social media influencer impacting people's habits.

In Australia, Jessica Ainscough was the original, self-proclaimed 'wellness warrior'. She was only twenty-two years old when she found some lumps in her left arm and had biopsies performed.[7]

In April 2008 she was diagnosed with a rare cancer called epithelioid sarcoma. She followed her medical team's advice and in June 2008 started chemotherapy. It looked like she was in remission, but when the cancer returned in November 2009, she didn't like what the doctors had to say.

She was told her best option for survival was to have her left arm amputated at the shoulder, but rather than heed this advice, she decided to take a different route and sought alternative treatments.

Under the supervision of a physician in Mexico, she commenced Gerson therapy – a supposed cancer cure invented in the 1920s that is ineffective and is not based on science. It involves taking lots of vitamins, minerals and enzyme supplements, consuming plenty of plant-based juices, and putting coffee up your backside five times a day – similar to what Belle Gibson was promoting around the same time.[8]

Jessica shared her journey with her online followers and amassed a community of 1.5 million people who were inspired by her battle against cancer. She appeared to sincerely believe in this ineffective treatment and rigorously participated in a regimen of drinking fresh juices and enduring coffee enemas multiple times every day. Unfortunately, her faith in the treatment was misplaced and she died in February 2015.

In their book *Lifestyle Gurus*, Dr Stephanie Alice Baker and Chris Rojek summarised this tragic outcome, saying 'all the evidence indicates that Ainscough acted from the best intentions', but 'the probability is that many cancer sufferers who followed her advice about conventional medical treatments are now themselves dead'.[9]

As a cancer researcher, Associate Professor Darren Saunders has plenty of experience speaking with people who have been diagnosed with terminal illnesses and understands why some people may choose an alternative to modern medicine. He explains, 'For many people, their experience of modern medicine is one of unmet expectations and profound disappointment.'

Medicine isn't perfect – it can't cure everyone, and it can't keep people living forever. 'When medicine runs out of answers,' Darren observes, 'a trust deficit creates fertile ground ... for false hope ... fake cures and conspiracies.'[10]

Wellness warriors may sincerely believe they are providing good advice but they can inadvertently mislead their audience if they are not formally trained in health sciences. They are often highly skilful at being approachable, entertaining and engaging, which makes it easy for their opinions on healthy living to be misinterpreted as fact.

Successful influencers are able to turn their wellness vlogs into a full-time business and over time their online presence can become distilled to a single goal – selling you stuff. Their personal lives become curated for the camera and whether or not they genuinely believe what they are saying or promoting, they can find themselves living in a giant advertisement selling a veneer of healthiness.

What worries me the most is our inability to differentiate fact from fiction. Social media influencers have a tendency to blur these lines, but unlike used car salesmen, real estate agents or politicians, we let our guard down and allow these online personalities into our lives without realising they are pushing products. What starts as a friendly face in a YouTube video ends up being a salesperson selling you cacao powder and leading you down a path in a perpetual pursuit of promised completeness.

Sarah may envisage she is 'helping' her audience by sharing personal anecdotes, lifestyle advice and information she has pieced together from her own experience. But this kind of helpfulness is like a toddler 'helping' you mow the lawn with a pair of safety scissors.

Influencers need to understand that their own unique perspective of the world doesn't give them the authority to provide health advice.

You might be thinking, 'Stop throwing shade at Sarah Stevenson. She's young and possibly a bit naive. What's the problem?'

The problem is that she has a large audience of impressionable young people, and with a big audience comes great responsibility. Medical experts have contacted her to raise concerns, but she ignores criticism.

This beautiful, bubbly and charming young woman appears innocent, but when she provides dodgy health advice to a massive audience, ignores feedback from health professionals and disregards the safety of her dedicated fans, we can consider her to be a menace to public health.

Sarah's day will come when her fans notice the danger she poses by preaching poor health advice and the blurred line she's created between opinion, advice and advertising.

●

So what lessons should health professionals and science communicators learn from savvy social media stars?

Associate Professor Darren Saunders has observed the techniques utilised by influencers and says that when it comes to communicating health messages, 'showing the human side of science is a very effective way of reaching entirely new audiences'.

He suggests that, 'Drawing on warmth, empathy and compassion helps people relate to us as humans.'

Unfortunately charisma isn't universal and academic lectures aren't commonly known to collect millions of views on YouTube or Instagram. Some health professionals and academics spend years researching hot health topics but are unable to communicate their knowledge in a way that's easily understood by general audiences.

Scientists need to replicate Sarah Stevenson's style of communication. Doing so will make it much easier to engage an audience online, relay important health information to a broader range of people, and be able to do this much more quickly and effectively.

Sharing medical knowledge in a more approachable, engaging and personable way will open up opportunities for health professionals to provide sensible evidence-based health advice.

Sarah Stevenson may not be listening to scientists, but scientists should be listening to her.

CHAPTER 6

THOUSANDS OF YEARS

After backpacking around the world in my mid-twenties, I returned to Melbourne but needed a change of scenery. The move to Coffs Harbour was specifically designed to give me a fresh start and hopefully improve my energy levels.

Travelling had left me with a hole in my pocket so I hunted out the cheapest accommodation in town – the local pub. It might have seemed a bit strange for the new doctor to rent a small room at the town drinking establishment, but I'd become pretty accustomed to cheap hotels and youth hostels so the facilities didn't bother me in the slightest.

My first-floor room had a stunning view of a brown-brick wall, but it was only a short walk to the beach. The only other hotel resident was an elderly man who briefly emerged from his digs twice a day to shower and brush his teeth in the communal bathroom. His hunched silhouette cast thin shadows against the faded walls, like the seaside town's version of Gollum.

I was committed to a six-month work placement at Galambila Aboriginal Health Service and still struggling to get through the day without copious amounts of coffee and a nap. Determined to avoid becoming the town's next Gollum, I hit the gym.

Living close to the beach meant I could go jogging along the sand every morning and having the clinic just around the corner meant I could duck home at lunchtime for a snooze. Achieving some sort of routine and work–life balance was possible, but my medical degree made me very aware that someone in their twenties shouldn't need a disco nap every day.

I slowly made friends in town and one day was introduced to a glamorous couple. She was stunningly beautiful and her boyfriend was a footballer with muscles on top of muscles and piercing blue eyes you could drown in.

He really only seemed able to talk about one thing – the science behind resistance training and weightlifting, so our conversations were filled with gym talk. One day he leaned up against me as he shared his secret. 'Do you want to know what gives me loads more energy?'

Of course the answer was yes. I nervously nodded for him to continue, as he whispered in my ear, his bicep pushing against my body.

'If you're serious about training, take what I'm taking,' he suggested. 'This stuff from the Chinese medicine shop on the main street.'

He didn't know what they were, or what they were called, only that they came in little black balls.

'Go into the shop and tell them you need an energy boost. He'll try to sell you some crap in a white package, but tell him you want the stuff under the counter. It's in a gold box. Trust me, you'll love it.'

Incense-filled rooms, mysterious herbs, dainty needles and healing massages are the immediate images conjured up when someone mentions traditional Chinese medicine, but I hadn't been taught much about this alternative way of healing at medical school. I knew that it was dangerous though. I had often seen patients admitted to hospital with anaphylaxis or liver failure after swallowing a mysterious elixir. To make things worse, the patients rarely knew what was in their concoction, causing confusion about the best treatment. My colleagues and I know to always check liver function when a patient tells us they have seen a traditional Chinese medicine practitioner.

However, desperation had set in. Western medicine hadn't found a cause for my fatigue, so again I found myself looking elsewhere – I had nothing to lose. Plucking up my courage, I strolled into the store and heard the echoing clink of the doorbell behind me. The shopkeeper peered up from his glasses and threw a questioning stare.

'Something to give my energy a boost?' I blurted out.

He nodded slowly and produced a white packet from the shelf behind him. 'No,' I politely declined, 'I've been told to ask for the gold box under the counter.'

The whites of his eyes widened and he stared back at me in suspicious silence. When he eventually reached down I became nervous, like I was about to get in trouble or a trapdoor was about to swing open beneath me and send me to a certain death. Instead he handed over a bright, shiny gold packet from his private cupboard.

Inside were a bunch of tiny black balls that looked remarkably like peppercorns. I turned the packet over to read the instructions and ingredients, but they were in Mandarin.

Later, back at the hotel, the 'medicine' stared up at me. I stood there in the bathroom pondering every permutation these pills could possibly provide. I thought about my new football friend's advice and wondered if I should take the plunge and swallow.

The palm of my hand was holding the future – an unknown substance of unknown potency.

'What will this do to me?' I asked myself.

My training as a doctor provides me with the ability to weigh up the benefits and risks of taking any registered medication – after all, we prescribe pills for our patients and expect them to trust us. We aim to provide patients with enough information to make an informed decision, but an inherent part of the process is conducting our own mental arithmetic to work out the pros and cons on their behalf.

Health professionals are quietly frustrated when patients don't take our advice, but holding those peppercorns in my hand gave me an insight into how patients must feel when they get home from the pharmacy with a new drug, open the packet and think, 'What will this do to me?'

The difference was that these weren't a registered medication, and no one had done the thinking for me. I had no idea what these pills would do – all I knew was that I wanted to feel better and this was an opportunity to break free from my pattern of exhaustion.

In retrospect I should have been more cautious, but I felt like I had nothing to lose.

I began with one, two, then three peppercorns each day. My energy improved. At the gym I was able to lift heavier weights and I was able to run faster along the beach. A midday nanna nap was still necessary, but my energy reserves were much better in the evenings.

I felt like they were having a positive impact. For the first time in a long time, I felt great. The pills made me happy and confident and gave me an extra bounce in my step.

Life was going really well, until I started to notice a subtle change in my mood. It became increasingly obvious that those little black peppercorns were making me hungry, horny and angry.

Vigorous exercise had likely dialled up my need for more calories, so I wasn't too worried about an increased appetite. An elevated libido was bothersome because I didn't have a partner at the time, but the anger was something else.

The little box of peppercorns was finished within a few weeks. While I had enjoyed the brief elevation in my energy, I was too concerned about my altered mood to invest in another golden packet.

The chemical cocktail contained within those little balls remains a mystery to me, but they appeared to act similarly to testosterone. The effect I experienced could have been caused by natural substances mimicking the action of male hormones, or the pills may have even been laced with synthetic pharmaceuticals. It's also possible that the placebo effect made me imagine the whole ordeal.

Unfortunately, it's impossible for me to know what I took because traditional Chinese medicine isn't regulated to the same extent as prescription medicine. I'm also lucky it didn't have any lasting detrimental impact on my health.

My infatuation with the handsome footballer lingered but I never had another opportunity to brush up against his bulging muscles, stare into his deep blue eyes or ask if he had noticed any mood changes from those tiny black peppercorns. The last thing I heard, he had pushed his girlfriend out of a moving vehicle.

●

Traditional Chinese medicine (TCM) has been used to treat multiple ailments for thousands of years, but just because something might have been used for a long time doesn't mean it works – or that it's necessarily good for you. It is one of China's major exports and pulls in massive profits. Use has exploded around the world in recent years, but as scientific researchers continue to methodically assess TCM, the results have been uninspiring.

The practices of TCM encompass a wide range of therapies including: herbs, acupuncture (inserting needles into the body), moxibustion (burning dried leaves near or on the skin), cupping (sucking skin to create bruises), tai chi (slow exercise), tui na (massage), gua sha (scraping skin) and qigong (exercise and meditation).

One of the biggest criticisms about TCM within the scientific community is that it isn't based on science.

This is hardly surprising as TCM was invented well before we knew practically anything about the human body. Most of it is based on the theory that vitalistic energy called 'qi' flows along channels called 'meridian lines' and different therapies are used to unblock meridians and enable this vital energy to flow more freely.

But this kind of 'qi' is a form of energy that has never been measured in a lab or even properly defined – and meridian lines don't exist.

Well-defined anatomical structures like blood vessels, nerves and even lymphatic pathways do not match up with the energy conduits our ancestors outlined. It may seem disrespectful to say they were wrong, but at the time they didn't know any better because their knowledge of human anatomy was limited. We know better now.

Traditional Chinese medicine practitioners might be charismatic and respected by their patients, but the education they receive is totally different from studying medicine. Many TCM practitioners claim they are able to identify different patterns of disharmony within the body and prescribe individualised remedies for each pattern of conflict. A diagnosis can apparently be made by observing the colour and shape of their patient's tongue, smelling their breath and listening to the quality of their voice. They may spend a long time palpating their patient's wrist and checking their pulse for characteristics described as floating, rapid, rough, replete, vacuous, string-like, sunken, surging, skipping, hollow or hidden.

These observations can be fairly subjective.

The radial pulse is definitely used in modern medicine to determine the speed and rhythm of the heartbeat. A range of anatomical pulse sites are also regularly assessed for the presence or absence of a pulse to check for obstruction of arteries, but TCM practitioners overreach its diagnostic capability.

It's impossible to diagnose problems with the liver, kidney or spleen from just touching a patient's pulse and a false diagnosis can cause significant health anxiety.

Patients have come to me totally convinced that death is imminent after their TCM practitioner palpated their pulse and diagnosed a 'stagnating liver'. Persuading patients that their liver is fine and they are not about to die can be difficult. It takes plenty of discussion, reassurance, a normal abdominal ultrasound and successive blood tests to alleviate their stress.

Most people expect to receive the same health outcome, whether they see an Eastern or Western doctor, but that's not the reality.

When you're buying prescription medication from your local pharmacy, you know it has been tested, standardised and gone through quality controls. Every batch is monitored to ensure you get the right dose of the right chemical, every time. Whether you're treating high cholesterol, low thyroid function or major depression, standardised health care and safe medical practices can assure you that you're getting the best possible treatment.

However, herbs and potions provided by TCM practitioners aren't regulated as stringently as pharmaceutical products, so you really don't know what you're going to get.

In 2015, a team from the University of Adelaide tested twenty-six different TCM products collected from the Adelaide markets. Multiple scientific techniques were utilised, including toxicology tests to detect pharmaceutical-grade drugs, mass spectrometry to detect heavy metals, and DNA analysis to determine the genetic origin of plant and animal material. A combination of these was used to identify the exact contents of each product, and then compared with the ingredients written on the label.

The results were shocking and showed that nine out of ten products contained a substance that wasn't listed as an ingredient. Half of the samples showed significant amounts of heavy metals, including arsenic, cadmium and lead. Some items even contained genetic material from cats, dogs, shrub frogs, rats, pit vipers, goats and snow leopards.[1]

I'm a massive fan of snow leopards, but I'm not keen for them to end up in my medication.

More surprisingly, some of these herbal products contained synthetic drugs made in an industrial laboratory. Paracetamol, antihistamines, anti-inflammatories, antibiotics, warfarin and even pseudoephedrine were found in these 'natural' TCM items – suggesting that these drugs were either added on purpose to create a therapeutic effect, or were accidental contaminants at the factory. Neither option is good and this lack of quality control is clearly dangerous.

We like to think only plants and herbs are used in TCM but the presence of endangered species like tigers, leopards, elephants, pangolins and rhinoceroses actually isn't unusual.[2]

Rhinoceros horn and pangolin scales are mostly made of keratin – the same protein that forms your hair, skin and nails. Keratin from exotic animals has long been touted as having healing properties but has never been proven to have any medicinal value. Yet even today their horns and scales are ground into powder and offered as treatment for health problems as variable as fever, infections, infertility, irregular periods, poor breast milk production, arthritis, liver disease and erectile dysfunction.

Consuming rhino horn or pangolin scales will give you exactly the same improvement in erectile function and period control as you would get from chewing your fingernails. There are better treatments so I'd prefer you do neither, but if you ever have to choose between biting your fingernails or allowing wildlife to be hunted to extinction, I'd rather you sacrifice your nails.

●

Herbal combinations are frequently used in TCM and it's claimed by some practitioners that it's the complementary mixture of plant material that provides the therapeutic effect. But from a scientific perspective it's important to know which compound is actually doing the heavy lifting.

Each herb can contain hundreds of chemicals and when multiple herbs are mixed together for a tailored TCM approach, thousands of chemicals might be administered at the same time. If the herbs actually make a real difference, it would be a pure guessing game trying to work out which one did what.

Modern science has purified many herbs used in TCM into single components and then tested each compound individually to see which one is the active chemical and which ones are filler, with mixed results. However, this approach isn't taken by TCM researchers.

A few years ago, I received an unusual phone call from a clinical researcher from a complementary medical facility asking if my patient was suitable for their trial. They planned to use TCM to improve sperm production in men and they wanted to know if there would be any anticipated problems if my patient took their product.

I asked the researcher what she planned to give my patient and learnt that the trial involved administering a combination of green tea, panax ginseng, grape seed extract, vitamin B6, vitamin B12, vitamin C, vitamin E, folic acid, cysteine, lycopene, selenium, co-enzyme-Q10, zinc, L-carnitine and acetyl-L-carnitine.

When she read out the list, I thought she was joking and asked which of these ingredients they were actually testing.

'Sorry,' she replied, 'but I don't understand the question. We're testing all of them.'

Since she was giving her patients fifteen ingredients simultaneously, even if she found a measurable improvement in their sperm production, it would be impossible to pick apart exactly what had made the difference.

The scientific process can be used to study TCM but poorly designed trials are not the way to do it. Research like this appears to approach the topic by assuming the herbs are going to work, and then goes about trying to prove it. This is opposite to the scientific method where you aim to thoroughly disprove your theory and if you don't succeed, you're correct.

The use of TCM over long periods of time doesn't mean these ancient treatments work – we could have just been fooling ourselves for thousands of years.

Let's look at the scientific evidence for some of the other common TCM practices.

ACUPUNCTURE

When I was studying human anatomy at university, I learnt the three-dimensional positions of various nerves and blood vessels as they wound their way from the spinal cord, around bones, muscles and tendons, reaching out to the fingertips and toes. After hours of staring at anatomy textbooks these pathways were firmly burnt into my retina, which is why my brain short-circuits every time I look at a meridian chart.

As discussed, vital energy called 'qi' is meant to flow along meridian lines and sticking acupuncture needles into various points along these lines is meant to encourage the normal flow of energy by unblocking them.

Doctors live and breathe human anatomy. We're constantly prodding and poking it with all sorts of surgical instruments and needles. Showing a diagram of acupuncture points to a medical doctor is like revealing a star chart of zodiac constellations to an astronomer. It looks familiar but doesn't mean anything tangible.

Similarly, we're also very familiar with human physiology and understand how the body transports and utilises energy, so we understand the concept of vitalistic energy flowing along meridian lines is incompatible with human anatomy and physiology.

However, it's not just TCM practitioners who make use of acupuncture. When I was accepted to study my Fellowship in General Practice I couldn't wait to start seeing my first patients. Training in Australia is set up with a mentoring system where your mentor is nearby whenever you need guidance or a second opinion.

My first mentor was absolutely fantastic, extremely knowledgeable and had an excellent rapport with his patients. One day I knocked on his door to ask a clinical question and opened it to find a bizarre scene.

A patient was lying prone on the treatment table and my mentor was hovering over them with a glowing wand-like device, like a wizard casting a healing spell. My bewildered expression was obviously apparent because he quickly explained that he was using laser acupuncture to treat his patient's chronic pain.

This was an everyday experience for my mentor, but it absolutely blew my mind. I was in disbelief that a GP with evidence-based training was flashing a fancy light at his patient's acupuncture points in an attempt to unblock their meridians. Acupuncture seemed like such an antiquated practice to me, he may as well have been cracking open his patient's skull to release their demons.

Laser acupuncture is a modern version of the old classic, where you're able to administer treatment without piercing the patient's skin or ending up with a bin full of sharp biohazard waste.

I started to wonder if I was being too judgemental. Maybe there actually was something in the ancient practice of acupuncture. Could this have been a blindspot in my medical education all along? I was certainly open to the idea and wanted to make sure I hadn't missed something important.

The Australian Acupuncture and Chinese Medicine Association is an organisation that provides information and training courses for health professionals in Australia. They justify acupuncture as a valid treatment option by saying that it originated more than two thousand years ago, making it one of the oldest therapies in the world.[3]

If acupuncture really works it will be able to stand up to the scientific method, but scientists have been arguing over the effects of acupuncture for decades. While plenty of trials say acupuncture works, plenty say it doesn't – so who can you believe?

In December 2019, Carole Paley and Mark Johnson looked at 177 studies examining acupuncture and pain relief published between 1989 and 2019. After trawling through all of these studies, they concluded that 'despite a high volume of published research' many of the randomised control trials had 'inconclusive findings due to persistent methodological shortcomings' that contributed to a 'high risk of bias and downgrading of evidence'. Essentially after decades of research there was no convincing evidence that acupuncture worked for relieving pain.[4]

Many of the trials that showed a positive effect actually had low numbers of participants, inconsistency in how acupuncture was being performed and/or inadequate placebo controls.

Therapists continue to debate the optimal ways of providing acupuncture. Opinions differ on the type and number of needles used, location and depth where needles pierce the skin, the needle technique of 'thrusting, rotating, flicking or pecking', and even how long needles are left in the patient. These kinds of inconsistencies between trials create a problem when you are trying to compare treatments.

Similarly there is no consensus about where on the human body acupuncture points are situated. Acupuncturists trained around the world will point to different positions on the body and locations will vary widely between practitioners.[5]

Lastly, being unable to use an appropriate placebo for the control group also leads to problems with interpreting data. If participants don't receive any needles, they'll know they are in the control group and this can affect their response.

Sham needles were created for exactly this purpose – to make these trials more valid. The end of the acupuncture needle is hidden from view so both the acupuncturist and patient are unable to tell if the needle has punctured the skin.

There's no denying acupuncture is fashionable and has become increasingly popular over the past few decades, but it may well be an elaborate, theatrical placebo itself.

Sticking pins in your back may not be doing anything to reduce your pain, but spending time lying down, relaxing in a quiet room and breathing aromatic incense could all be providing the therapeutic effect, rather than the needles.

The practice isn't totally benign, however. There are cases around the world where patients have required major surgery to fix a problem that's been caused by the practice.

Needles inserted into the chest and particularly near the clavicle (collarbone) only need to penetrate a few centimetres before piercing the fragile pleural layer sitting around the lung. This can cause a pneumothorax (punctured lung) and you will quickly move from the relaxing acupuncture room to the emergency department and possibly surgical theatre.

There are reports of acupuncture needles penetrating the heart, liver, kidneys, spleen and major blood vessels. Acupuncture needles have even caused cellulitis and sepsis after bacteria that was sitting innocently on the skin's surface was accidentally injected into the subcutaneous fat.

The idea that you might have to have major surgery or require months of intravenous antibiotics seems like a high price to pay for using a therapy that is unsupported by evidence and likely gives no better benefit than a placebo.

MOXIBUSTION

Moxibustion is the process of burning herbs like mugwort near acupuncture points in an attempt to unblock meridians and improve energy flow. Smouldering herbs are either held close to the patient's skin or attached to the end of acupuncture needles.

If acupuncture itself can be described as a theatrical placebo, then adding smoke and fire can only increase the theatre, but not the therapeutic effect. It's also more dangerous. Burning dried plant material close to your body significantly increases the potential to cause harm – it's not just the risk you'll suffer a burn, but inhaling smoke can also trigger asthma or other respiratory problems.

There's no scientific reason or studies to explain how moxibustion could possibly work. You may as well stand in front of a campfire and unblock all your meridians at once – at least you'd be able to toast some marshmallows at the same time.

Moxibustion has traditionally been used for health conditions including chronic pain, high blood pressure, ulcerative colitis, cancer and to hasten recovery after a stroke, but a systematic review performed in 2010 couldn't find enough evidence to support its use for any of these problems.[6] However, the researchers outlined one condition they felt deserved further attention – flipping babies.

In the late stages of pregnancy, babies usually prepare for a vaginal exit by changing from a head-up to a head-down position. Cephalic presentations (head-first) are far less risky than breech presentations (bottom-first), so it's common to feel more anxious about the delivery day if your baby isn't aiming in the right direction. Moxibustion has historically been recommended as a way to turn babies up the right way, but it's hard to imagine how burning mugwort near the tip of your fifth toe is meant to encourage an intrauterine somersault.

In 2012 a thorough review of the evidence was performed and moxibustion wasn't found to have any effect on a breech presentation.[7] But even though this therapy has been completely debunked, rumours will persist and heavily pregnant women will continue to singe their toes.

CUPPING

I, like most Australians, love cheering for the green and gold at the Olympics. I've also been known to celebrate the wins of my Kiwi homeland too, when no one is looking.

But I distinctly remember being outraged by the US swimming team's 'secret weapon' back in 2016.

As their champion, Michael Phelps, pulled himself out of the water everyone could see he was covered in circular bruises. I told the media at the time that it looked like he'd lost a fight with a vacuum cleaner.

The circular suck marks were from cupping – a practice where glass cups are heated and placed directly onto your skin. Cupping is meant to help blood pump more freely to the area and draw out toxins – but it doesn't. It's got just as much therapeutic value as a giant hickey.

A vacuum is formed within the cup, sucking up the underlying tissue. Fragile blood vessels become dilated from the negative pressure and this enables more blood to flow into the area. Increased blood flow sounds like a good thing, but not with cupping. The blood vessels are put under so much strain that they pop and blood leaks out into the surrounding tissue.

Toxins aren't released because the blood doesn't go anywhere – it's trapped inside your body as a giant circular bruise, doing as much good for your health as walking into a door.

It isn't an effective treatment and it's certainly not safe.[8] Heating up glass cups and applying them directly to your skin can cause terrible burns and make patients look like freshly branded cattle with permanent circular scars.

The risk of burn injuries can be reduced by using plastic instead of glass. Hard plastic cups are placed on the patient's skin with a tube attached to a suction device. Air is pumped out of the cup, creating negative pressure over the skin. This method might prevent burns but it doesn't completely prevent injury. Too much negative pressure can cause massive blood blisters to form, which can take forever to heal and the stagnant blood they contain can become infected and require antibiotics.

'Wet' cupping can be even more dangerous. This is when the skin is punctured before applying the cups in an attempt to suck out 'bad blood'. Unfortunately the cups aren't able to differentiate between good and bad blood, so they just suck out blood. Sometimes the suction is so successful that the cups fill up to the brim with thick blood clots. Puncturing the skin is risky because any break in this protective barrier creates an entry site where bacteria can get in.

Cupping isn't effective – in fact, it leaves some people with deep bruises, blood blisters, strange-shaped scars and even life-threatening cellulitis. But it is popular. It's popular because people like Michael Phelps, Sonny Bill Williams, Jennifer Aniston, Justin Bieber and Kim Kardashian show off their bruises to the masses, giving the treatment credibility among fans.

TAI CHI AND QIGONG

When I was younger, I never understood the point of tai chi and qigong. I liked the general idea of learning martial arts but thought the movements would be way too slow to win a fight.

Now that I'm a little bit older, I'm able to comprehend how tai chi and qigong could possibly be the most useful and well-tolerated therapies out of all TCM.

Exercise isn't always about slogging it out at the gym or building up a sweat. Slower exercise can be used as a form of relaxation and can alleviate stress. Gentle exercises are unlikely to cause harm, which makes them safe for people of all ages, helpful for people recovering from injuries and another option for rehabilitation.

Bone density decreases with age and osteoporosis has become a major problem in our elderly population. Reducing falls is a major priority and these slow exercises can improve balance by boosting muscle strength, enhancing muscle tone and increasing flexibility.[9]

While tai chi and qigong may not help you fend off an attacker it could prevent you from falling over and breaking a hip.

•

Traditional Chinese medicine covers a broad range of treatments. Some may be helpful, but most have the potential to cause harm. Some of these therapies have been normalised to the point that registered health practitioners, even doctors, administer them to patients.

But we need to think rationally – all medical treatments need to be based in science and evidence. Facts don't care about tradition.

CHAPTER 7

TWEAKING, BOOSTING AND RATTLING

Every few months I have patients come to me with concerns about being on prescription medication long term. One such patient was Patty, who arrived at the clinic one day to complain about feeling rundown. Unfortunately, she hadn't been coming in for regular check-ups, and when I asked whether she'd been taking her meds, her response was one I'd heard before.

'I stopped about eight months ago,' Patty revealed. 'I started taking multivitamins instead.'

It turns out she'd swapped her thyroid medication for vitamins, and then the tiredness had set in not long after. I asked if she thought there might have been a connection.

Patty thought carefully, 'I suppose I thought I'd try something a bit more holistic.'

I understand the concerns that many people like Patty have, but all the vitamins in the world wouldn't have helped her feel better. Unsurprisingly, her energy level did return to normal once she started taking her tablets again.

The thyroid gland sits at the base of your neck, acting as an internal body clock. When your thyroid is overactive, your metabolism speeds up. When your thyroid is underactive, your metabolism slows down.

Once your thyroid stops working, it generally doesn't come back to life and Patty's thyroid stopped functioning a few years ago. It wasn't producing enough thyroid hormone to keep her body happy and the pills are what brought her levels back to normal.

No one wants to take prescription medication every day, but people like Patty need to. Even if she dramatically improved her diet and made significant lifestyle changes, she would still feel terrible if her thyroid hormone wasn't topped up properly.

Prescription drugs aren't always the answer, though. For example, in the early stages of type 2 diabetes you're likely to get greater health benefits from lifestyle changes, increasing physical activity, improving your diet and losing weight than you are from just popping a pill. But if you've made these changes and your blood sugar level keeps going up, then medication becomes a necessity.

Despite this, it can still be a battle convincing patients to go on regular medication, especially if they believe anything 'natural' must be better for them than what a doctor can prescribe.

Not long after my experience with traditional Chinese medicine, I became intimately acquainted with the pharmacy shelves that Patty had been frequenting when she gave up her prescriptions.

Vitamins, minerals and supplements come in a range of colours, flavours and purported benefits. I was willing to give anything a go to beat my constant exhaustion, especially if the packet promised higher energy or better sleep – and, like Patty, I was attracted to the idea of a natural solution.

Vitamins are one of the most common 'natural' alternatives people choose to take.

Unfortunately, they don't help balance your thyroid hormones, and randomly picking supplements off the shelf is generally a waste of time and money. For unwell people this action will only delay appropriate care or make you feel worse, like Patty.

The rational part of my brain knew that if my vitamin levels were normal I wouldn't get any benefit from taking a multivitamin, but I felt like I was running out of options. A decade of my life had been spent going from coffee shop to coffee shop to get through each day.

I needed an energy boost, so I tried whatever I could get my hands on – vitamin C, B group vitamins, vitamin D, fish oil, krill oil, glucosamine, andrographis, silica, echinacea, probiotics. If someone had given me a good shake, I would have rattled.

Doctors don't like running out of ideas. It's frustrating to reach the edge of evidence-based medicine and find ourselves staring into the abyss while our patient still needs help – it's even more frustrating when you're also the patient.

My own GP at the time must have felt this pressure too, so they offered me vitamin B12 injections. They explained that anecdotally they'd seen some patients get a lift of energy after the injections, so we decided to give them a go. Vitamin B12 is unlikely to be harmful, it's relatively cheap and there was a slim chance it could be helpful.

I remember asking what to expect, 'Will I see results tomorrow or in a week?'

The response was quick, 'Oh, with the patients I've seen, they usually get an energy boost straight away.'

I was impressed, 'What kind of patients have you seen this working on?'

'Horses,' the doctor replied. 'I used to work with race horses and they'd get tired travelling long distances between competitions. We'd bring them out into the field and they'd be sluggish, so we'd draw up a big dose of vitamin B12 and inject it into one of the veins in their neck. It worked wonders! They'd immediately start sprinting around.'

If someone approached me and stabbed my jugular vein with a needle, I'm sure I'd start sprinting around the track too. Thankfully, my doctor only injected the vitamin into my arm, but I didn't bounce or even trot out of the clinic. After three weeks of regular injections, I wasn't feeling any better, so we gave up on the idea.

High dose vitamin B12 injections have been given to patients with low energy levels for decades, especially in people diagnosed with chronic fatigue syndrome, but studies haven't shown they work any better than a placebo.[1]

Of course, if you're deficient in the vitamin you'll feel much better after a shot – but if your fatigue isn't due to low B12, giving super-high doses won't fix the problem.

The same principle applies for other vitamins. If your doctor diagnoses you with a deficiency you'll get benefit from taking a supplement, but when your vitamin level is already normal it won't do you any good.

I went back to caffeinated drinks.

VITAMINS

The word 'vitamin' was initially coined by a biochemist with one of the best names in the world. Casimir Funk was born in Poland in 1884 and worked in Switzerland as a biochemist where he combined the words 'vital' and 'amine' to become 'vitamin'.

Vitamins are 'vital' for our bodies to work effectively. We can't produce them ourselves, so we need a steady supply from an external source, our food. Amine is the name given to chemicals derived from ammonia, and when Casimir Funk discovered the initial vital amines, he found they all had similar molecular structures that contained ammonia.[2] Researchers subsequently discovered more chemical compounds in our diet that are also vital but don't contain ammonia, but the word vitamin had already stuck.

We now have a list of thirteen vitamins essential for human life: vitamin A, B (eight of them), C, D, E and K.

We haven't stopped pumping them into ourselves since they were discovered. But whether you're taking vitamin tablets, capsules, injections or attending a fashionable wellness clinic for an intravenous infusion, they probably won't do you any good if you don't have a deficiency.

Deficiencies caused by an inadequate diet are rare in Australia because we generally have access to healthy food. When your vitamin levels are within an appropriate range, you'll hit that sweet spot where your metabolic processes are working like a well-oiled machine. But if your body becomes saturated with an abnormally high concentration of vitamins, you'll overshoot – adding more oil to a well-oiled machine doesn't make it go any faster.

B group vitamins and vitamin C are water-soluble, which means that once your body has used the vitamins it needs, any excess is filtered through your kidneys and eliminated in your urine. Your body isn't able to store them for long and you need a steady supply trickling in through your diet; however, they're generally considered to be safe, even at high doses.

Vitamins A, D, E and K are fat-soluble, which means your body can store a supply within your fat cells and drip-feed it back into your system when necessary. You can survive for long periods of time without needing a regular dose of these vitamins in your diet, but excessive amounts build up and become toxic. Vitamin toxicity can cause liver failure, loss of vision and even death – so more isn't always better.

People living with conditions like inflammatory bowel disease, short gut syndrome and chronic diarrhoea might not absorb enough nutrients through their intestinal wall, requiring regular top ups. Also, some prescription medications will decrease the amount of available vitamins, for example Methotrexate (an immunosuppressant) requires regular supplementation of vitamin B9 (folic acid).

Pregnancy places a huge nutritional demand on the body, so supplementation is generally recommended. Neural tube defects (problems with the spinal cord developing) can be minimised by taking folic acid for a few months prior to getting pregnant and throughout the first and second trimesters. Extreme morning sickness during pregnancy (hyperemesis gravidarum) can cause significant vitamin deficiencies, and multivitamin supplements – especially vitamin B6 (pyridoxine) and vitamin B9 – are recommended.

Your gut may not absorb vitamins very well in your senior years, but you can tell if you're deficient by having a simple blood test. The vitamins most likely to be low in this situation are vitamin B12 and vitamin D.

Rare genetic conditions can cause problems with absorption and transportation of vitamins around the body, and these require specialised care. There are some rare forms of epilepsy where children can benefit from large doses of vitamin B6, but this needs to be administered under close supervision of a paediatrician.

Unless you fall into one of these specific categories, you probably won't benefit from taking vitamins.

●

There is probably no other figure in Australia who feels more passionately about the widespread use of vitamins, minerals and supplements than Associate Professor Ken Harvey. He has spent many years of his career as a public health physician examining not only the scientific evidence behind using supplements, but also looking at their promotion, regulation and use in this country. He told me, 'There are far more beneficial phytonutrients in a healthy diet than in any multivitamin/mineral pill.'

Yet more than a third of Australians take dietary supplements every day, and about two-thirds of Australians take supplements occasionally.[3]

'The usage of these vitamins and supplements is out of proportion to the evidence to support them,' Ken told Jenny Brockie on the SBS current affairs program *Insight* in March 2019.[4]

I asked Ken why vitamins and supplements are so popular in Australia and he told me it is 'a triumph of celebrity endorsement and hype over science. If you look at the advertising, which is enormous, that has an effect.'

But why do so many Australians spend money on health products they don't need? Ken says the answer is 'because industry lobbying is strong, and the TGA is weak'.

The Therapeutic Goods Administration (TGA) is Australia's regulatory authority for health products and therapeutic goods. One of their roles is to keep Australians safe by ensuring health products sold in the country are made to an acceptable standard and that they're okay for human use. They also regulate the advertising and therapeutic claims made by companies about their products.

Prescription medication goes through a rigorous process to assess its safety and effectiveness, but these quality controls aren't in place when it comes to dietary supplements. There are fewer checks and balances, and instead a trust-based regulatory system is in place, which relies on companies to do the right thing by their customers.

In Australia, companies selling over-the-counter health products must register the item with the TGA via an online form. They are asked to supply information about their product and pay a fee to the TGA, but it's not a requirement for the product itself to be tested before it goes onto the shelf for sale.

The TGA relies on companies to tell the truth and monitor their own products, but this self-regulating system doesn't offer much assurance that the product is safe, will effectively treat your health problem, or even that you're going to receive the ingredients written on the box.

Relying on these companies to do the right thing through a trust-based self-regulatory system seems outrageous.

The TGA might do a great job when it comes to regulating prescription medications, but over-the-counter products regularly make it onto the shelves even if their health claims are misleading or deceptive.

John Skerritt, the head of the TGA, shared a studio with Ken Harvey on that episode of *Insight*. He was keen to point out that the TGA performs post-marketing surveillance, where products have their health claims assessed – but this is only conducted after the products have made it onto the shelves.

John tried to be reassuring, explaining that every year about eleven thousand new products start being sold over the counter in Australia and post-marketing surveillance is performed on a few hundred of them. This is really a phenomenal statement to make – it stopped me in my tracks. Sell first. Ask questions later. Sometimes.

John continued by saying, 'We don't check [the evidence] for every medicine because resources simply don't allow it, so we do a mixture of targeted and random reviews.'[5]

Ken expressed on *Insight* that testing only some of the products reaching Australian shelves wasn't good enough. He also noted that eighty per cent of the products chosen for surveillance failed the test because companies didn't have evidence to support the health claims made.[6]

In response to this criticism, John replied 'What's most important, however, is safety, and the products can only contain ingredients that are shown to be safe and they have to be produced within a medicines-grade facility. Australia's got the strictest safety requirements in the world.'[7]

It's great that our regulator has a primary focus on safety and on providing high-quality ingredients, but products should also deliver the benefits they promise.

If the TGA allows Australians to buy high-quality, safe nothingness, then they are missing the point. At the end of the day, are these vitamins and supplements actually effective and giving people benefit, or are people just wasting their money on products that don't do anything, and forgoing products that do?

Our consumption of vitamins, minerals and supplements is driven by clever marketing strategies rather than scientific evidence. We're given the impression that if we feel stressed, start to get crook or want an energy boost, then a handful of vitamins will help us out. Eating too much junk food can make us feel guilty, but instead of improving our diet we appease our guilt by topping up with supplements. They're seen as an insurance policy, but they can distract us from addressing our original health problems and poor diet.

In 2020 Australians spent over five billion dollars on complementary and alternative medicine products.[8] This money isn't being spent wisely unless the intention is to support the profits of supplement companies.

Our healthcare system could do with an extra five billion dollars each year, but most of this money is going straight down the toilet.

VEGETABLES, FRUITS AND SPICES

It's not just vitamins that people believe are a healthy alternative to prescription medication. Vegetables, fruits and spices are commonly bottled up and used for a variety of ailments.

Garlic

Garlic has a health halo around it. If you've ever eaten a raw clove of the stuff, you know it makes you feel like your sinuses are opening up and your head is going to explode. Something that leaves such a strange aftertaste must be good for you, right?

Garlic is believed to heal all kinds of health conditions including hypertension, heart disease, common colds, and some people even tout it as a cure for cancer. Incredible health benefits were originally said to be present when it was added to your food, but now it's also sold as a dietary supplement in tablets and capsules.

I had a patient enter my clinic recently after not seeing a doctor for about ten years. He had a feeling that something wasn't right with his health and wanted a bit of a once-over. I examined him – his health wasn't too bad, except his blood pressure was extremely high. It was sitting at 210/140, when a healthy blood pressure is less than 135/85. Over many years, blood pressure at this level will place significant strain on the walls of your arteries and increase the risk of having a heart attack or a stroke. Since my patient hadn't seen a doctor in over a decade, I presumed his blood pressure had been elevated for a long time.

High blood pressure, also called hypertension, is known as a 'silent killer' because it can be there for years without causing symptoms, then suddenly you have a heart attack, a stroke or die.

His blood pressure remained consistently high throughout the consultation. I was eager for him to start taking medication to get him out of stroke territory, but he wasn't interested in taking tablets.

I made a deal with him – he would see me again in a week's time and if his blood pressure continued to be elevated, then he would start medication.

Even though I was feeling on edge with his blood pressure so high, I also knew it had most likely been chugging along at this level for years. Another few days shouldn't be a problem.

He attended the clinic the next week and arrived earlier than his allocated time. He was happy to wait to see me, but my receptionist wasn't. I got a call from her soon after he walked through the door, asking me to see him straight away. As he entered my room, I immediately understood why.

A common survival skill for GPs is to politely ignore noxious odours, but it was difficult to keep a straight face without gagging. He absolutely reeked.

The stench lingered in my nostrils while I checked his blood pressure again and he revealed that he had been trying to reduce his blood pressure 'naturally'.

Between shallow gasps I asked what this involved and he said he had heard that garlic was good for blood pressure, so he had been eating lots of it. I initially thought this meant he had been adding more garlic to his spaghetti bolognese, but he clarified that he didn't have time to make Italian meals and had just been eating eight cloves of raw garlic each day.

The smell permeated out of every bodily orifice and crevasse. I tentatively read his blood pressure and it was still a resounding 210/140 – it hadn't budged one iota.

He thankfully admitted that his garlic treatment must not be working and was willing to try my plan instead – prescribed medication that wouldn't cause those around him to wilt.

While this is just one anecdotal story (and my patient only took garlic every day for a week), what does the actual evidence suggest?

In 2014, a systematic review was published in the *American Journal of Hypertension*, looking at the effect of this bulbous plant on blood pressure. The researchers identified nine relevant trials that used garlic supplements compared to a placebo. There were 482 participants in total for a period of at least eight weeks. In the end there was a small decrease in blood pressure for patients taking garlic, but the evidence wasn't strong. A mild effect of lowering blood pressure might help some people, but when your blood pressure is through the roof garlic supplements just aren't enough to reduce your risk of a stroke.[9]

Cinnamon

Some of my patients take supplements to assist their prescription medication rather than replace it. Like Lisa, who was having trouble getting on top of her sugar levels. She had already seen the diabetes specialist and was taking tablets and insulin but wanted to know if there was more she could do. She thought cinnamon could be the answer.

I've mainly had cinnamon on donuts and other delicious desserts, but sugary treats aren't the best option if you've got diabetes. However, cinnamon capsules are available over the counter to give you a large dose without the extra calories. As long as she was still taking her other medication and allowed me to monitor her progress, I didn't have a problem with her giving it a go.

Fluctuating blood sugar levels can be a problem for some people living with diabetes. An average blood glucose level is between 4 and 8 mmol/L. Sugar levels higher than 11 mmol/L are toxic and start damaging small blood vessels and nerves around the body. Hypoglycaemia occurs when glucose levels drop below 4 mmol/L and makes people feel dizzy, weak or faint. Patients need urgent medical attention or they collapse and end up in a coma.

As you can see, balancing out glucose levels to keep them in the Goldilocks zone is important – but cinnamon isn't the answer.

In 2019 a systematic review found eighteen studies relevant to cinnamon and diabetes management. The overall result suggested that cinnamon supplements made a modest improvement to a patient's morning blood glucose level. But it's more complicated than that.

Blood glucose levels are only a snapshot in time, but there is another blood test called HbA1c which gives you a big picture view of your blood glucose over a three-month period. Even though cinnamon may have marginally improved the morning blood tests, an overall improvement of HbA1c just didn't happen.[10]

The HbA1c test is a great way to determine how diabetes management is going and, like the subjects of the systematic review, my patient found cinnamon supplements didn't improve her HbA1c either.

Small doses of cinnamon are unlikely to cause any problems, but high doses can damage the liver. My patient's liver function was fine but she did notice some other side effects – stomach cramps and diarrhoea. She decided it wasn't worthwhile continuing.

Severe health problems can be tricky to manage, even for the most well-trained doctors and vigilant patients. Dietary changes, regular exercise and medication when necessary will give you the best control of your diabetes, but relying on cinnamon to treat a severe case is like trying to put out a bushfire by pissing in the wind.

Cranberries

One of the first home remedies I heard about as a young medical student related to the treatment of bladder infections. I was taught that any patient presenting with symptoms should drink cranberry juice three times a day.

We were told that the juice provided an inhospitable environment for bacteria in the bladder and helped people get better more quickly.

Years later proanthocyanidins (PACs) were identified as the special compound in cranberry juice that attached to the lining of the bladder wall and made the surface slippery.[11] Bacteria wouldn't be able to establish an infection because it wouldn't be able to latch onto the wall of the bladder.

This gave doctors more confidence when recommending cranberry juice to our patients, but we were also taught some new information – if you already had a bladder infection it was too late for cranberry juice to help. It would only work as prevention, so patients with recurrent infections were advised to drink cranberry juice every day.

But it turned out it wasn't that simple.

In 2012 a Cochrane review pooled together data from 4473 participants over twenty-four studies. Even though some of the smaller studies suggested cranberry juice helped reduce the number of bladder infections, when all the data was compiled together, no statistical difference was seen between the control and treatment groups.[12]

Basically, they didn't find that cranberry juice decreased the number of bladder infections. Importantly they also found that plenty of people couldn't stand drinking cranberry juice every single day.

Further complicating matters was a later study published in *The American Journal of Clinical Nutrition* in June 2016. Regular consumption appeared to reduce the frequency of bladder infections in women, but the results were subtle. The study concluded that you would need to drink cranberry juice every day for more than three years in order to prevent one infection.[13]

That's a huge amount of juice, but before you go out and buy enough to last the next three years it must be noted that the study was criticised for having a potential conflict of interest – it was funded by a company that sells the stuff.

Also in 2016 a randomised control trial was published that tested high dose PAC capsules against a placebo. One hundred and eighty-five women living in nursing homes participated, all of whom were considered to be at high risk for developing urinary tract infections. The number of recurrent infections was not statistically different between the PAC and placebo groups over twelve months.[14]

So, now we're facing an interesting quandary that tends to occur all too frequently in science and medicine.

Early trials showed some benefit; a systematic review didn't show any; a further trial tested the compound suspected to be responsible and this was negative too; and in conclusion everyone continues drinking cranberry juice in a misguided attempt to prevent bladder infections.

Based on the evidence, it would make sense for everyone to stop drinking their daily glass – but that's not what has happened. Rumours persist and people get stuck in their ways – many are already in the habit of regularly drinking the juice, doctors are used to recommending it, and cranberry juice companies are able to advertise using the cherry-picked studies they like.

Ginger

When I was a kid my grandmother used to give me ginger beer whenever I had a stomach-ache. Ginger has historically been thought to have medicinal qualities and used to calm down nausea, digestion issues and diarrhoea. Nana might have been onto something because some research does suggest that ginger can be helpful when it comes to decreasing nausea and vomiting, but not so much for diarrhoea. However, you would need to consume it at much greater levels than what I was having in my ginger beer.[15]

But sometimes the cure can be worse than the disease. Ginger in high doses can cause a reaction in some people's delicate digestive systems resulting in abdominal pain, heartburn, diarrhoea, bloating and flatulence.

Ginger can also accumulate in the gut and may interact with prescribed medications, preventing them from working. It's certainly not a panacea for gastrointestinal issues, but it may be helpful in moderation for some people.

Fish Oil

One of the most revolting studies I've read over the years came from New Zealand in 2015 where researchers acquired a variety of common fish oil capsules, cut them open and examined the contents. They found that eighty-three per cent of the samples contained rancid oil that had oxidised over time.[16]

Doctors have been recommending fish oil capsules to patients for years in an attempt to prevent heart attacks and stroke, but recent research has been disappointing.

In 2018 a meta-analysis examined the data from ten trials with more than 77,000 patients and concluded that daily fish oil capsules might alter your cholesterol profile, but didn't show a reduction in the number of heart attacks, stroke or any other vascular disease.[17]

Fish oil was thought to lubricate osteoarthritic joints, and some guidelines even recommended for patients to take nine to fourteen capsules every day for osteoarthritis, but research hasn't shown a major improvement when compared to a placebo.[18]

Fish oil capsules are one of the most popular supplements sold in Australia, but the benefits are now seen to be dubious when the oil is fresh, and ingesting rancid oil is very likely to cause you harm.

Turmeric

Turmeric is a mild spice known for having anti-inflammatory properties. It's so popular that you've probably seen turmeric lattes on the menu of your local trendy cafe and fancy restaurant. Curcumin has been identified as the active ingredient found in turmeric, which is available in tablet or capsule form and sold on supermarket and pharmacy shelves all over the world.

While it is true that turmeric has been shown to have anti-inflammatory properties in a controlled laboratory setting, results from human trials have been disappointing. Your body struggles to absorb it from your gut, and once it has been absorbed, it doesn't last long – it's only in your bloodstream for a few hours before your body gets rid of it, which doesn't allow much time for it to have a therapeutic effect.

In an effort to counter this problem, higher and higher doses of curcumin have appeared on our shelves, but increased doses don't improve the anti-inflammatory effect. It's still poorly absorbed, so you're only going to increase the severity of side effects, including abdominal pain and diarrhoea – which may distract you from your knee pain, but isn't a great solution.

Resveratrol

Everyone has heard that a glass of red wine is good for you. It's an oft-repeated myth that people use to justify the extra glass late at night. Resveratrol is the antioxidant responsible for this claim. Found in the skin of grapes, blueberries, raspberries and most famously red wine, rumours of its anti-ageing effects started spreading widely in the 1990s.

But further research identified there was so little resveratrol in red wine that any attempt to drink enough of it would be dwarfed by the harmful effects of alcohol.[19]

High-dose resveratrol pills started popping up as a solution to this red wine dilemma, but yet again research found that even high doses of resveratrol provided just as much youthfulness as a placebo.[20]

The resveratrol craze died down, but this hasn't stopped it from being sold over the counter, nor used as an excuse to crack open another bottle.

Raw Milk

Some people like the idea of natural products so much that they forgo some of the safety features built in to the systems we use for food production and distribution.

In late 2014 a three-year-old boy died and a number of other children around Australia suddenly became sick. These kids all had one thing in common – they had all been drinking the same brand of raw milk, straight from the cow's udder and into a bottle with being pasteurised.[21]

The product had been distributed to health food stores and markets around the country as 'bath milk' with labels stating the milk wasn't for human consumption, but instead should only be bathed in.

Raw milk can be dangerous and can't be sold in Australia for the purposes of drinking.

It is generally okay to drink if it's extremely fresh, described as having a creamy, full flavour that's significantly different from the milk you buy from the supermarket shelves. Fans claim it contains more nutrients, is better for people with lactose intolerance, and suggest it helps prevent allergies in children.

You'll probably be okay if you live on a dairy farm or if you live in the city with your own cow standing there, ready to go, in your kitchen. But if you don't live within close proximity to your own milky teat, then things can get a bit dicey.

The problem is timing and transportation.

Transporting milk from the farm to your home can take a considerable amount of time if you live in the city. The untreated version contains a small amount of bacteria when it comes out fresh – so small that it's generally not enough to make you sick. However, as the milk is transported and time passes, the bacteria in the milk grows exponentially. As the clock ticks from pasture to person, your raw milk could end up containing dangerous amounts of deadly bacteria, and people do occasionally die from drinking it. High doses of campylobacter do not make a healthy milkshake.

Louis Pasteur is the reason the milk you buy at the supermarket is safe to consume. He discovered that heating it up to a moderate temperature could destroy the bacteria it contained, without obliterating all the nutrients. His method of pasteurisation changed our diets forever as milk could be transported safely around the country without fear of bacterial contamination or the death of unsuspecting customers.

The pasteurisation process might slightly alter the flavour, but safety is key. Most people are happy to sacrifice the supposed additional creaminess for a product that will let them and their families live to see tomorrow.

Raw Water

Raw water advocates are not dissimilar to raw milk fans. They believe the chemical processes and filtration techniques used on our public water supply are introducing unnecessary toxins and are keen for everyone to drink from rivers and streams so we can all reap the benefits of 'natural' water.

Unfortunately, the quality of water is variable depending on the time of year, speed of water flow, and whether or not a dead sheep is decomposing upstream.

Most people would understand the danger of drinking untreated water. Anyone who has had a case of 'Bali belly' when visiting our neighbours to the north would be thankful for the modern filtration systems we have in place in Australia.

Raw water proponents are generally quiet. Every now and then you'll hear them start to protest, but they are unable to get many people to agree to drinking water from an unknown source.

PROBIOTICS

We've known about gut bacteria since the mid-1600s when Antonie van Leeuwenhoek took samples from around the body, placed them on his microscope and began documenting the tiny 'animalcules' he saw writhing around on a glass plate. Despite this, almost four hundred years later, we're only now starting to scratch the surface when it comes to understanding the impact our gut microbiome has on our general health.

It wasn't a major topic when I was going through medical school, we were mainly taught about the wicked pathogens that could cause profuse diarrhoea.

This is no longer the case – we're slowly unravelling the mystery contained within our intestine, but we've still got a long way to go.

This isn't the impression you get when you walk through pharmacies and health food shops today. Over two hundred probiotic supplements are now available in Australia, many of which claim to hold the secrets to gut health, prevent bladder infections, stop diarrhoea, and even boost your immune system. Fridges and shelves are full of probiotic capsules, powders and yoghurts, with expensive price tags to go along with them.

Your gut microbiome has been described as being like the rainforest spread across South America. Just as the rainforest contains a variety of river dolphins, sloths, macaws, anacondas, capybaras, anteaters and jaguars, your microbiome is also extremely diverse with different types of bacteria.

One probiotic capsule containing seven billion bacteria might sound like a lot, but when your body harbours approximately a hundred trillion bacteria, it sounds less impressive.

Taking one capsule of seven billion lactobacillus each day would be like adding a hundred cloned butterflies to the Amazon rainforest. First of all, you're unlikely to impact the whole rainforest. Second, if you happen to add the wrong species, you could inadvertently harm the local ecosystem. And third, once you stop adding butterflies, they'll get gobbled up by the other rainforest animals and disappear.

Some people experience irritable bowel syndrome and find repetitive episodes of diarrhoea, constipation and abdominal cramps debilitating. In these cases, sometimes probiotics are recommended by health physicians, but this treatment is generally a stab in the dark.

We're slowly starting to understand that a healthy gut microbiome is more about the diversity of bacterial species rather than simply ingesting a single type of bacteria. For people with tricky bowel issues, it's best to seek advice from a gastroenterologist who is up to date with the latest research, rather than taking a lucky dip at your local pharmacy or health food shop.

•

It's tempting to buy vitamins and supplements. It's a multibillion-dollar industry, easily accessible, and has advertising that's targeted and pervasive. But I can't overstate the benefit of simply eating good food. If you're otherwise healthy, consuming a wide range of vegetables in your diet will supply you with all the vitamins your body needs.

If you are taking vitamins or supplements, take in a list to show your doctor on your next visit. Many people don't realise that some supplements have the potential to interact with prescribed medication, can alter results of some pathology tests and could inadvertently be causing you harm.

Health professionals are generally happy to assess what you are already taking, rationalise your medication, check for interactions and work out a plan for the future.

When you find yourself wandering down the aisle of your local pharmacy, reaching for a bottle of tablets, ask yourself if you really need them. Calculate how much you're spending each month on supplements and work out if your money would be better spent on healthy food, a gym membership or a pushbike.

CHAPTER 8

QUACKS

When I first heard the term 'alternative medicine', I was confused.

I'd trained hard to become a practitioner, so why would someone actively seek out an alternative practitioner – what's so appealing about an alternative me?

Adapting Josh Thomas's words of wisdom outlined at the start of this book – when your car needs to be fixed you don't seek out an alternative mechanic. You'd feel uneasy if you discovered an alternative electrician had wired up your house. And I think we'd all find it hard to place our lives in the hands of an alternative pilot.

What could have gone so wrong in modern medicine that patients would look for an alternative?

Whether you call it alternative, complementary, holistic, integrative, or any other name used as a branding exercise, the practice of combining unproven remedies with modern medicine is widespread and sneaking into our lives. Naturopathy, applied kinesiology, iridology, traditional Chinese medicine, homeopathy and acupuncture appear to be credible because they are taught at tertiary institutions alongside evidence-based subjects and courses.

Therapies that have previously been debunked persevere as part of the curriculum of our highest educational facilities. It should be a national outrage. But education is a business, and as long as enough unsuspecting people are willing to hand over money to be taught fictional ideas, teaching establishments will continue to provide these courses.

Same goes for those who actually attend an alternative medical practitioner or buy ineffective items that populate our pharmacy shelves and the healthcare aisle of our supermarkets. Many of us pour cash down the drain buying expensive treatments that do us no good – but why?

It often comes down to three factors – trust, fear and a patient's circumstance.

TRUST

Every now and then patients can have bad experiences with doctors. We're all human, so personality clashes happen, and while health professionals can be experts, sometimes you just don't click.

A negative interaction can erode the trust a person has in the medical establishment.

When you're feeling sick and needing assistance, you're also bound to be feeling anxious. People are already on edge – throw in a delay in treatment, poor communication, or the sense that problems aren't being appropriately addressed, then your anxiety level will go even higher.

It only takes a second to become disillusioned and lose confidence in your treating physician.

As discussed, when I was attending my family clinic as a teenager with a bone tumour in my back, the GP initially scanned the wrong area of my body, gave me the wrong diagnosis and sent me for treatment that only caused more pain. I can understand how a bad experience with one doctor could make you distrust others and even turn away from modern medical care completely.

But as a GP, I know it can be difficult to immediately ascertain the correct diagnosis, and the remedy needed to treat it. Health issues can be complex and sometimes present themselves more clearly over time.

Another reason some people come to dislike doctors is because we frequently deliver bad news – there's rarely any sugar coating. As a doctor, there have been plenty of times when I've needed to give patients bad news. There's no easy way to tell someone that they have metastatic cancer, multiple sclerosis or will never be able to walk again. It's not fun for anyone in the room. Telling the truth, warts and all, is what we are trained to do. It can be frightening to receive a poor diagnosis, but sometimes instead of focusing on the diagnosis itself, people can turn their anger to the messenger.

It can be easier to be angry at a person than a tumour, but these are not good reasons to turn away from lifesaving treatments.

If you don't hold complete confidence in your doctor, you need to get a second opinion, but choosing to see an alternative practitioner instead can be disastrous.

FEAR

When I worked in the hospital, one of my jobs was to run the cardiothoracic surgery pre-admission clinic, preparing patients for major heart surgery. They looked healthy enough on the outside, but on the inside their hearts were withering away.

I'd need to explain to patients in very simple language that we were planning to use a general anaesthetic to put them to sleep, we'd then cut through their sternum to get into their chest, and stitch veins from their legs onto their heart to bypass the blocked arteries.

It's no wonder patients are frightened to have modern medical treatment when we do such weird and wonderful things to them.

When your options are laid out in front of you and you have the choice to either have major heart surgery or do nothing and die from a massive heart attack in the next few months, most people will take the risk of surgery. But many alternative therapies offer hope, free of that overwhelming fear of surgery.

CIRCUMSTANCE

Our cultural, spiritual and religious backgrounds all influence the way we think about illness and disease, so it makes sense that people are more likely to seek out healthcare solutions that align with these beliefs. Plus our family and friends will often suggest practitioners they believe in, and we're more likely to trust them if they come highly recommended – even if they aren't evidence based.

We're also restricted to our physical location and finances. If we live in a remote area and can't get an appointment with the appropriate specialist nearby, then we'll seek an opinion elsewhere. If we're unable to afford to see the best person for the job, we'll find someone more affordable – even if they point us in the wrong direction.

Humans do what they must and make do with what they've got.

NATUROPATHY

I like to think of naturopaths as the ringleaders of the alternative medicine world. They amalgamate a wide range of pseudoscientific ideas into their diagnostic and treatment repertoire, not only misinforming their patients, but often misinforming themselves too.

They aim to provide holistic care with a personalised, tailored and natural approach to healing that relies on the use of fresh air, water, sunlight and healthy diets. They also use iridology, reiki, homeopathy, and recommend a range of vitamins, minerals and supplements.

They believe in the healing power of nature and the body's natural ability to fix itself when provided with a healthy environment.

I don't believe naturopaths knowingly give out poor advice to patients, they may truly think they are doing good. But diagnosing people using unreliable tests, offering unproven or disproven treatments and discouraging patients from accessing modern medical care is misguided and can be dangerous.

APPLIED KINESIOLOGY

Kinesiology is a legitimate study of human movement, but applied kinesiology is a whole different kettle of fish. Practitioners claim they can diagnose illnesses by testing muscle movements for weakness. The first time I heard of the practice was during a simple medical consult with a new patient when they told me they were allergic to milk.

A proper allergic reaction to cow's milk protein could cause a rash, wheeze, shortness of breath or anaphylaxis. However, lactose intolerance is different – it's often described as an allergy but is actually caused by not having enough lactase enzymes in the gut. Your intestine is unable to metabolise lactose sugar contained within milk which can give you diarrhoea, bloating, abdominal cramps and flatulence.

My patient wasn't sure which affliction milk caused, only that their applied kinesiologist diagnosed them, and that they hadn't had a bowl of cereal in years.

Food allergies and intolerances are usually diagnosed by an allergist or gastroenterologist – and it's an involved process.

A sample of blood might be sent off to the lab for a RAST test (radioallergosorbent test) where we can look for specific IgE antibodies associated with a milk protein allergy.

Alternatively skin prick testing might be used. This technique involves dipping the end of a small needle into a solution containing the protein you're interested in. Your skin is scratched with the end of the needle and an allergy to that particular protein is diagnosed if the surrounding area becomes inflamed.

Lactose intolerance is even more involved and requires a gastroscopy with biopsies taken from the intestinal wall. These small samples of tissue are checked for the presence of lactase enzymes and if low numbers are present, that means you'll likely have trouble metabolising the lactose in milk and spend a lot of time on the toilet.

My patient didn't have any of these tests. Instead their applied kinesiologist asked them to stand on one leg with both their arms held out horizontal to the ground. The practitioner then pushed down on the patient's forearm, asking them to stay upright. The experiment was then done again, but this time with the patient holding a small flask of milk. The second push resulted in him falling over.

The applied kinesiologist told him that holding the milk had made his muscles weak, which was why he had fallen, ergo he was allergic.

I was flabbergasted.

Milk trapped behind the walls of a flask will not interact with the body and make one's muscles weak.

When we discussed it logically, my patient was able to realise that when they went shopping and collected a bottle of milk from the supermarket fridge, they were able to carry it around with the same muscular power as they did a bottle of orange juice.

The fall is caused by the practitioner pressing on the arm while also subtly pulling the arm away from the body and combined with the ideomotor phenomenon. The ideomotor phenomenon is when you have an expectation of a result and your brain surreptitiously and unconsciously alters your muscle movement to favour the result you're expecting. This can happen to both the practitioner and the subject.

The practitioner expects a patient to be allergic to milk (or any substance) and then unknowingly pulls the body in such a way to get the desired outcome. In the end, they feel they are genuinely performing the test with an innocent, unbiased attitude, but behind the scenes their brain is working towards the outcome they are expecting.

The subject can also complicate the situation by having their own expectations.

Unfortunately this convincing magic trick can give people the wrong diagnosis, and therefore can significantly impact their health.

Patients who have been diagnosed with food allergies by an applied kinesiologist will alter their diet accordingly. Some may feel better if they make healthy changes, but it's dangerous to unnecessarily ask someone to exclude major food groups.

Patients have come to see me at the clinic extremely worried about their liver, pancreas or adrenals because they've been told by an applied kinesiologist that they have a problem. We'll perform blood tests and conduct ultrasounds to examine their internal organs only to find that everything is completely fine. Valuable time and money are wasted just to reassure people.

A 2015 review of alternative therapies by the Commonwealth Department of Health set out to determine which ones should be covered by private health insurance companies. It found there was no clear evidence that the practice of applied kinesiology was effective.[1]

GERSON THERAPY

Earlier I mentioned Jessica Ainscough, the original wellness warrior, who turned to Gerson therapy in an attempt to cure her cancer. The practice was named after Max Gerson, the German doctor who came up with the therapy in the 1920s.

He created a strict wellness regimen to treat his migraines, and after he found it worked for him, he decided to share his untested therapy with the rest of the world. If he were around today, he'd have a very popular Instagram following. However, Gerson therapy is ineffective for most health problems it claims to treat, including cancer.[2]

It involves three regular practices: an organic vegetarian diet with fruit and vegetables that contain high concentrations of potassium and low levels of sodium; vitamin, mineral and enzyme supplements; and enemas that contain coffee or castor oil.[3]

The whole theory is based on an incorrect assumption that people with cancer have too much sodium and too little potassium in their bodies. Consuming organic fruit and vegetables, in combination with juice drinks, is supposed to restore the balance. Multiple coffee or castor oil enemas are meant to remove toxins from your liver and colon, and vitamins, minerals and enzyme supplements are said to kill off your cancer cells.

Preparing, juicing and drinking raw organic fruit and vegetables is time consuming and this therapy quickly becomes hard to swallow, especially as the protocol often recommends drinking juice every hour. Add to this the unpleasant and messy task of pouring coffee or castor oil up your backside and it quickly loses its appeal. If I only had a few months to live, it's not how I would choose to spend my remaining days.

Gerson therapy hasn't been shown to cure cancer but does give you a sore bum. It has a large following around the world, but many people who choose this path of treatment unfortunately don't achieve anticipated longevity.

HOMEOPATHY

Unlike me, my friend Lizzy had never had a problem with falling asleep. But work had been stressful, and she was spending her nights staring at the ceiling mulling over the events of the day. Until she found a miracle remedy in her local pharmacy. Only four drops of it under her tongue worked wonders, and she started sleeping like a baby.

I was fascinated to hear more about it, until she showed me the bottle. It was homeopathic – the only active ingredient was the power of her active mind.

Homeopathic products come in a liquid form with a dropper or a spray bottle to put the liquid under your tongue, or as sugar pills with the homeopathic solution dripped onto individual tablets. They do not contain any active ingredients and these placebos are often sold in health food shops and pharmacies, sitting on the shelves beside legitimate products. Their positioning in such locations lend them a credibility they don't deserve, and people often pick them up by accident.

Lizzy had been using a placebo, which was fine for her as she was just needing to treat a lack of sleep. Not so fine if you're trying to treat a more serious issue.

The therapy was established in the eighteenth century by a German physician called Samuel Hahnemann. Honestly, this was a time before scientists really had a great grasp of medicine.

Hahnemann's theory was that 'like cures like'. For example, if you have insomnia and coffee keeps you awake, then tiny doses of coffee would make you go to sleep. But when we're talking tiny doses – I mean really tiny.

There are two main classifications for diluting homeopathic substances, 'C' and 'X'.

Take one drop of coffee and add it to ninety-nine drops of water and give it a shake. That's a 1C dilution in homeopathic terms. Take one drop of this watered-down coffee, add it to another ninety-nine drops of water and shake it. That's a 2C homeopathic dilution. Do this thirty times and you'll have a 30C dilution and a very weak cup of coffee – so weak that you may not even have any of the original drop of coffee left in your mixture.

A 1X dilution is a similar process, but one drop of coffee is instead added to only nine drops of water, and so on.

These solutions resemble water much more than coffee, but Hahnemann theorised that as an active ingredient gets increasingly watered down, it gets stronger.

I suppose if you hadn't heard of homeopathy before, you'd be wondering how it is actually meant to work.

Well, the secret is apparently succussion.

Succussion is the fancy name for shaking the solution by repeatedly hitting it against a surface. This process is meant to activate the original ingredient and allow it to disperse its memory into the rest of the surrounding water or alcohol it has been diluted in.

Homeopathic products are cheap to produce and clearly profitable but are no better than a placebo – it's daylight robbery.

Some proponents of homeopathy suggest if it's just a placebo, then it couldn't possibly cause any harm, but choosing to take homeopathic products can delay receiving appropriate medical care. The longer some health problems are left untreated, the more difficult they are to manage.

Homeopathic vaccines are another dangerous product found on the shelves. Pretending to immunise someone against a potentially lethal infection by using a placebo vaccine is deceitful and can be deadly.

In 2015 the National Health and Medical Research Council (NHMRC) reviewed all the available scientific research and concluded there was no reliable evidence that the therapy was successful.[4]

OXYGEN THERAPY

Towards the end of my medical degree, I picked up a part-time job at a hospital in Melbourne as a pathology collector, taking blood from patients. Every lunchtime, one of my phlebotomy colleagues would tell everyone he was ducking off for an oxygen break. He would lay down on one of the beds, tuck in some nasal prongs and give himself oxygen for about half an hour.

He told us it would improve his skin and make him live longer, but it's not proven to do either.

Oxygen bars and clinics offering oxygen therapy have gone in and out of fashion for many years, selling expensive air – sometimes even flavoured. Practitioners who offer this service usually claim it reduces stress, improves concentration and mood, and increases energy levels – but these claims have never been proven.

Oxygen is transported from the air you breathe, across the lining of your lung and into your bloodstream. Normal room air contains twenty-one per cent oxygen and this concentration is high enough to saturate ninety-nine per cent of your haemoglobin molecules.

Haemoglobin picks up oxygen and moves it around the body, like a bus picking up and dropping off passengers. Increasing the concentration of oxygen in the air is like adding more passengers to the bus stop but doesn't make the bus bigger or add more buses. When the bus is already at capacity, there's nowhere for extra passengers to go.

Administering oxygen can be lifesaving during a medical emergency like altitude sickness, pneumonia or a heart attack, but recreational oxygen when you're healthy and breathing properly won't do much.[5]

For my colleague, making the decision to quit cigarettes would have assured more longevity and fewer wrinkles.

IRIDOLOGY

The coloured part of your eye is the iris, and it's as unique as your fingerprint. The practice of iridology is based on reading the colours and flecks of your iris to predict and detect disease.

However, your iris doesn't change all that much over your lifetime, which is why it's difficult to comprehend how iridologists could possibly diagnose a new disease from a stable structure.[6]

Legend has it that Hungarian physicist Ignatz von Peczely came up with the therapy. As a child he apparently broke the leg of an owl by accident. As he nursed the owl back to health, he noticed a black fleck in its iris fade. Associating iris discolouration with fractured bones seems like a loose connection. It's much more likely that he injured the owl's eye at the same time as he injured its leg.[7]

Iridology is essentially like palm reading but using your eyes instead of your hands.

REFLEXOLOGY

Reflexology is based on the theory that meridian pathways carry energy from specific areas of your feet to particular internal organs, and if you massage just the right spot, you'll be able to enhance the flow of energy to the corresponding organ.

We've already discussed how meridian lines were made up before we knew much about human anatomy. They have never been proven to exist, so relying on them to improve the function of your organs seems a bit unrealistic.

I am totally up for a foot massage though, as they can be pleasant and relaxing – but don't be fooled into thinking it's going to perk up your spleen.[8]

REIKI

I met Gus on a bus when I was backpacking through South America. You never know who you're going to meet as you travel through Peru, but Gus was a lovely American guy who was also travelling solo. Gus and I started talking about health problems we'd encountered during our holidays.

When you're in the middle of nowhere and hiking up huge Peruvian mountains, you really don't have much medical support nearby. When you're in your early twenties you also don't have that much disposable income to spend on pesky things like your health.

I told Gus about the birthday gift I gave myself: a yellow fever vaccination in Miami. He told me how he had healed his middle ear infection in an isolated town on the side of a mountain.

Gus had been staying at a youth hostel when his left ear started to ache. The pain and deafness increased in intensity just as he was about to start the first leg of a three-day hike.

Cue panic.

Luckily another backpacker at the hostel offered a treatment – reiki.

With no medical service nearby, and running out of options, he accepted her offer.

She asked him to close his eyes, put his shoulders back and relax. After she placed her hands near his ears, he felt a warm sensation across his face, gradually the pain disappeared and with a sudden 'pop' his hearing came back. He didn't have any problems during the hike and had been fine ever since. He was convinced her incredible reiki hands and healing energy had worked a miracle.

The origin of reiki can be traced back to a Japanese man called Mikao Usui in the 1920s. While on a twenty-one-day retreat of fasting and meditation he heard voices that gave him 'the keys to healing', although with hindsight it must be noted that anyone starving themselves is likely to begin to experience delirium and auditory hallucinations.

Reiki is composed of two Japanese words, 'rei' meaning 'universal spirit' and 'ki' meaning 'life energy'. This form of energy healing is based on the theory that energy flows through the body in a way that science can't explain and that by placing hands close to – but not touching – the body, the life force can be altered and the flow of energy can be improved.

In a nutshell, reiki practitioners state that they are able to harness the energy of the universe and channel it through their hands, passing it into another person. They use this in an attempt to heal a number of medical conditions, including mental health problems, pain and sometimes even cancer.

So what happened to Gus?

After discussing it further I came to the conclusion that he probably had a blocked eustachian tube, with fluid unable to drain from his middle ear – a common problem at higher altitudes. Sitting upright and relaxing his jaw may have opened up the tube enough to allow his ear to drain, resulting in the sudden 'pop' with a decrease in pressure and pain.

Mystical healing energy used to quickly dissolve bacteria associated with a middle ear infection seemed far less likely.

There are three, sometimes four, levels of reiki practitioner. The first level can be achieved in a single session by having another bestow the universal energy into your body after placing their hands around you.

I myself happen to be a level one reiki practitioner. Many years ago, when sitting around a campfire I was asked whether I wanted to be filled with reiki energy so I could heal other people with my hands. I pointed out my profession already allowed me to do so, but was then told it would serve to enhance my healing potential – and who wouldn't want that?

My campfire friend placed their hands near my body for a few minutes. I could feel parts of my body become warm, which I was told was due to the healing energy flooding into me. In retrospect, it was probably partially from the campfire and partially me blushing from embarrassment. And, after a few minutes, I could add this qualification to my résumé. So I'm now officially able to use reiki to treat myself, friends, family and animals, but only within close range.

It takes a bit more effort to become a level two practitioner, which allows you to heal people by using reiki from a distance, through the use of phone calls, video calls, or at your own convenience – after such a session you can send your patient an email to tell them it's been done.

The training for levels three and above is much more involved. I haven't continued my studies or attended any more campfire lessons because there's no scientific proof that any of these energy fields around the body exist.

SPINAL MANIPULATION

Some people love getting their back cracked, but others shudder at the thought. Nevertheless, everyone seems to have an opinion about who is the best person to see when you've got a backache.

There is a significant crossover in the treatments offered by physiotherapists, chiropractors and osteopaths.

Physiotherapists have a reputation for basing their treatments on science and evidence. They are able to assess your physical issue, provide a diagnosis and teach you how to fix it, while taking your past medical history, current level of activity and hobbies into account.

Physiotherapists are more likely to use active therapies as treatment, where you are encouraged to move and strengthen your muscles in a structured exercise program. They focus on helping you help yourself and will usually give you a number of exercises to do between sessions.

In the early stages of treatment your muscles can be stiff and tight, so passive therapies like deep tissue massage can be used to improve flexibility and mobility of joints. They'll occasionally use joint mobilisation or manipulation.

Physiotherapists also specialise in different areas, such as rehabilitation to help patients recover after a long period of illness or an operation, chest physiotherapy to assist patients with breathing difficulties, and pelvic physiotherapy to strengthen a patient's pelvic floor and improve continence.

Osteopaths use both passive and active treatments. This includes deep tissue massage, joint mobilisation, spinal manipulation therapy and encouraging an exercise program to strengthen muscles.

Osteopathy was first conceived by Andrew Taylor Still in 1874, based on a principle he came up with that diseases are caused by pressure on nerves and blood vessels, and could be cured by spinal manipulation.

In Australia, osteopathic training is very different from medical training as it mainly focuses on spinal manipulation and back health. However, in the US there is a fair amount of crossover between medical doctors and osteopathic doctors because some of their medical schools started off training osteopaths before merging to also teach medicine.

Chiropractors are known to focus more on passive treatments with an emphasis on spinal mobilisation (pushing a joint to its limit) and spinal manipulation therapy (pushing a joint to its limit and then a little bit further till it 'cracks').

They occasionally provide physical exercises to do for homework as part of an active treatment regimen. Some chiropractors provide dietary advice and a few have been known to discourage vaccinations – which is worrying.

But when it comes to actually cracking your back, does it work?

The act of spinal manipulation involves moving a joint to its natural limit and then thrusting until you hear it crack.

A systematic review of the therapy was published in the *British Medical Journal* in 2019, showing that the practice provided a slight improvement in function when compared with using a placebo for acute low back pain, but no significant effect for chronic low back pain.[9]

But there is ongoing debate in the medical world regarding the benefit versus risk of having spinal manipulation performed.

Low back pain is common and if there are no red flags to signal something more sinister, then an episode generally gets better within a few weeks if you keep active.

Still, people choose to crack, which could be dangerous. In 2017, John Lawler visited a chiropractor in Northern England for a third session of chiropractic treatment after being diagnosed with shoulders that were out of alignment. During the manipulation the eighty-year-old complained he couldn't feel his arms and then his body went limp. His neck had been broken and he died the following day.[10]

In 2018, a 32-year-old woman in West Virginia underwent chiropractic manipulation, during which she developed a tear in her vertebral artery, a major artery in the neck. This caused a stroke in her brainstem and she died soon after reaching hospital.[11]

Cases like this may seem rare, but they are common enough that many emergency departments follow standard diagnostic protocols as soon as they hear a patient has seen a chiropractor.

The risk of a vertebral artery dissection, subarachnoid haemorrhage (bleeding on the surface of the brain), paraplegia, dislocation of cervical vertebrae, stroke or death is small, but I would much rather my patients avoid the risk altogether.

There is also the issue of chiropractors making claims that they can treat health problems that don't seem to relate to the spine.

When chiropractic treatment was invented by teacher Daniel David Palmer in 1895, he believed we have a life force called 'innate intelligence' which flows through our nerves and that when our spine is out of alignment it restricts our nerves, disrupting this energy flow and resulting in disease.[12]

His 1910 teaching guide on the subject, *Text-book of the Science, Art and Philosophy of Chiropractic for Students and Practitioners*, claimed that 'ninety-five per cent of diseases are caused by displaced vertebrae; the remainder by laxations of other joints'.[13]

The theory was that all of these diseases could be easily treated by correcting the alignment of the spine, alleviating the pressure on nerves and allowing the innate intelligence to flow freely again.

There's no evidence to support such claims.[14]

In fact, there's an ongoing debate between doctors and chiropractors about the use of the term 'vertebral subluxations'. Doctors refer to vertebral subluxations as a significant displacement of one vertebra in relation to another that can clearly be identified on an x-ray. These subluxations cause nerve damage or paralysis if the spinal cord becomes squashed.

Some chiropractors use the same term to describe a problem they can detect when performing a physical examination of a patient. They may find in their assessment that some vertebral joints are slightly out of alignment or inflamed and causing pressure on the nearby nerves. However, the changes they say they can feel during an examination are often unable to be seen on any form of medical imaging – making it difficult to confirm a diagnosis or monitor if a treatment is working.

Chiropractors split into two groups – straight practitioners who closely follow Daniel David Palmer's teaching, and mixed practitioners who employ a range of treatments including massage therapy.

Some people feel incredible after attending their chiropractic session, like everything has been cracked back into the right place. Others end up with a vertebral artery dissection, a tear in the covering around their spinal cord with a cerebrospinal fluid (CSF) leak, or a stroke. Some chiropractors ask their patients to attend every week for quick 'adjustments' that might only take seconds to perform. This is where they claim to correct subluxations that we can't detect with imaging.

Chiropractors have also been known to crack the backs of newborn babies and these videos are horrifying to watch and hear. Many doctors like myself take umbrage with chiropractors treating young children.

In 2016, Melbourne chiropractor Ian Rossborough was seen to perform spinal manipulation on a four-day-old baby in an attempt to treat infantile colic. This prompted the Royal Australian College of General Practitioners (RACGP) to advise against referring patients to chiropractors.[15]

In 2019 a shocking video appeared online of another chiropractor manipulating the spine of a two-week-old baby. In the clip he held the small child upside-down by the legs and was seen to use an 'activator' to strike the child's tailbone, neck and spine and then repetitively tap the baby on the head.

The chiropractor, Andrew Arnold, and the child's parents appeared calm throughout the video, but the baby cried throughout.[16]

The Victorian Health Minister at the time, Jenny Mikakos, found the footage 'deeply disturbing' and called for the Chiropractic Board of Australia and the Australian Health Practitioner Regulation Agency to take action. She also instructed Safer Care Victoria (SCV) to undertake an independent review of the evidence for and against spinal manipulation in children to ascertain if there was actually any benefit for what looked like a barbaric treatment.

The SCV report was completed in October 2019 and their recommendations were eloquently prefaced, saying it wasn't easy to come to a conclusion either way. 'To say that the lack of strong evidence of either effectiveness or serious harm failed to provide robust foundations for recommendations would be an understatement.'[17]

As they were unable to find convincing evidence of chiropractic treatment being helpful but were aware of the potential to cause harm, the final report recommended that spinal manipulation 'should not be provided to children under 12 years of age, by any practitioner, for general wellness or for the management of the following conditions: developmental and behavioural disorders, hyperactivity disorders, autism spectrum disorders, asthma, infantile colic, bedwetting, ear infections, digestive problems, headache, cerebral palsy and torticollis.'

Like any profession, there are good and not-so-good practitioners. As discussed earlier, as a teenager I attended weekly appointments with an osteopath for six months and they didn't help at all. Serendipitously, I saw a locum osteopath who was able to put his finger on the diagnosis straight away.

If you're seeing any of these therapists, be very wary of neck cracking – it can do more harm than good. And be careful if they offer to treat your kids, especially newborn babies.

ROGUE DOCTORS

Of course this chapter must include those rogue medical doctors who arguably have the potential to be the most dangerous of all our quacks. These are people educated in evidence-based medicine, who for whatever reason cease to use their critical brains and instead abuse the trust of their patients.

Patients like my Nana, who I remember telling me a disturbing story many years ago.

Nana was pretty tough. She left home when she was fourteen years old, lived through World War II, and raised five children while her husband was either away with work or at war. There were many reasons why she might have felt rundown, but apparently her medical doctor told her it was all due to 'sprays'.

She was advised that her tiredness was due to pesticide poisoning from the local council spraying her neighbourhood and that she needed to build up her tolerance.

I recall her saying he would place a small drop of pesticide under her tongue on each visit, causing her to feel terrible for the next few days. She believed this meant the treatment was working and would allow her to tolerate the pesticides sprayed around her neighbourhood.

She fortunately lived to a ripe old age, but I still wonder what damage those chemicals did to her body over the years.

I'd like to tell you that all doctors will give you great advice, but this isn't always the case.

Every profession has cowboys.

CHAPTER 9

SLEEPY DEMONS

Years of feeling exhausted had taught me that I needed to manage my day carefully; I'd set three alarms for the morning so I wouldn't miss work, I'd rarely be seen without a coffee cup in my hand and I'd try to take a quick kip during lunchtime at my clinic.

My perspective of what was normal had shifted.

A friend recommended I see her housemate who was a naturopath. I was reluctant, but one day at a party as I went to pat a gorgeous poodle, the naturopath cornered me for over an hour.

She told me I clearly had adrenal fatigue – my adrenal glands had supposedly run out of puff and couldn't keep up with my stressful life, which made me tired but too anxious to sleep at night. She was so confident that vitamins and ginseng would do the job that she offered to see me without charge at her naturopath clinic (with a free acupuncture session too), but I politely declined.

Around the same time, I was concerned when my GP told me he had pretty much run out of ideas. Until one day, unsure what to do with me, he asked whether I'd ever had any weird experiences while sleeping.

The answer was yes.

When I'm actually able to drift off, I'm pretty much dead to the world – albeit with an overactive dream life. It takes a lot to rouse me, but I've been told I frequently talk, shout or act out my dreams, kicking any unfortunate person trying to sleep next to me.

I shared the story of the time my sister locked herself out of the house when I was a teenager. On this particular night she arrived home late and I was fast asleep. Her constant knocking didn't wake me up, nor did the incessant barking of Ziggy, our Cavalier King Charles Spaniel. After scoping out the house, she and her boyfriend found my bedroom window was open, managed to pull off the fly screen and climb through the gap, landing on my bed in the process – with me in it.

Still, I didn't wake up.

They got the fright of their lives and I peacefully slept through the whole ordeal. When I got up in the morning, the window was wide open with the fly screen on the ground outside – I thought we'd been robbed.

It's not normal to sleep through a burglary, even when it's your own family performing the break and enter.

My GP was intrigued and asked if I had a history of fainting or falling over during times of extreme stress or emotion.

The answer again was yes.

There have been a number of occasions over the years. There was the time I fainted during a blood test, and the time I passed out while being berated by my mother for bleaching my hair.

Plus, there was my history of general clumsiness – bumping into walls, stumbling over and repeatedly dropping my pen at the end of a long day. At parties I'd even need to steady myself against tables when someone told a funny joke. I'd always assumed my blood pressure was low, but my doctor told me that was unlikely to be the case.

'That was probably cataplexy,' he told me. 'It's time to send you to a sleep physician.'

It was the first time anyone had suggested the cause of my exhaustion could actually be sleep-related. Cataplexy is a weird symptom where your muscles suddenly relax during times of extreme emotion, commonly associated with narcolepsy.

The sleep physician organised for an overnight sleep study, followed by a mean sleep latency test. The overnight sleep study was as predicted – my usual insomnia at the start of the night, followed by very active dreams and fragmented sleep throughout the night.

In the morning I was woken up early and asked to stay awake for two hours. Then the technician would tuck me back into bed, switch off all the lights and leave me alone to see if I was able to doze off. After fifteen minutes, if I was asleep she'd wake me up to start the two-hour cycle again.

The average person will find it increasingly difficult to fall back to sleep as the day continues, until the afternoon when they generally don't fall asleep at all.

The technicians didn't let me drink coffee, so the two hours between naps were a struggle – I was forced to pace the room just to keep alert.

When my results came in, they showed I was able to reliably fall asleep within four minutes.

The results were conclusive. My night and daytime sleep pattern was consistent with narcolepsy.

It was news to me. I didn't really know much about narcolepsy apart from what I'd seen in the movies – people falling asleep mid-conversation or while standing up. They were often the butt of a joke or not taken seriously. Unfortunately, I hadn't learnt anything about narcolepsy or cataplexy at university or even during my general practice training.

I quickly learnt that this sleep disorder has been described in literature and depicted in classical artwork for centuries. The most typical feature is a feeling of exhaustion and tiredness during the day, followed by insomnia when you're trying to get to sleep at night.

Your circadian rhythm is completely out of alignment, and your brain might as well toss a coin to decide whether it should be awake or asleep.

Vivid dreams are common, with hypnagogic (as you're falling asleep) and hypnopompic (as you're waking up) hallucinations – a blurred border between sleep and being awake. A car alarm down the street might be incorporated into your dream or characters from your nightmares might feel like they follow you into your waking hours.

Sleep paralysis is also common – waking in the middle of the night, frozen in place. Lying in your bed, you might be able to look around the room, but you're unable to move any other muscles. It's usually accompanied by the strangest sensation of foreboding, like there is an evil presence in the room, sometimes it's sitting on your chest.

These odd experiences were very familiar to me. I've spent many conversations describing my movie-length dreams in great detail to others, only to have them look confused and perplexed in response.

I've also felt unable to move when I've just woken up. I originally thought I was being attacked by demons but explained it away as an extension of a dream.

It's only recently that medicine has been able to confirm the cause of these extreme symptoms.

It was only in the late 1990s when we discovered that narcolepsy occurs in people with a poor production of orexin (or hypocretin).

The reason I felt so exhausted for so long was because my brain wasn't producing enough of this wakefulness hormone. My body was in a constant state of confusion, not knowing whether to be awake or asleep, so it sometimes did both.

It was life changing to realise that my experience was real. I hadn't been making it up; I wasn't just needing to suck it up and get over it. I had truly been struggling for years. I had finally found a diagnosis and the cause of my troubles.

It all made sense.

I was privileged to be given the opportunity to turn my mind to managing my condition properly and to look beyond simply surviving each day.

The treatment is relatively simple. A tiny dose of an old-fashioned antidepressant stopped the nightmares, night terrors, sleep paralysis and demon visitations in the mornings. It also gave me the ability to sleep through the night without waking up every few minutes.

Stimulant medication during the day helped me stay awake and alert. Topped up with well-timed naps, I was a new man.

After years of seeing multiple doctors, quacks and trialling all kinds of vitamins, supplements, teas, meditation, Chinese herbs, lifestyle and diet changes, the answer was finally delivered from evidence-based, Western medicine.

There wasn't a cure, but there was an answer. And it's so much easier fighting a battle when you know the name of your enemy.

Narcolepsy with cataplexy is such a niche diagnosis that it took the skills of a senior sleep physician and a complicated diagnostic test to eventually solve my medical mystery.

No amount of vitamins or ginseng were ever going to solve this issue. Seeking advice from a naturopath would have only been another distraction. I would have had more success talking to the poodle.

CHAPTER 10

SEXIST MEDICINE

It would be fair to say that, historically, women have been treated poorly by the medical establishment – this isn't surprising since doctors were once exclusively men. As a result, the male body is always thought of as the norm when treating health issues.

Medical trials predominantly recruit more men than women even though there are considerable differences in size, shape, metabolism, medication side effects and life experiences between genders.

The health profession has traditionally assumed that female patients are just feminine versions of men. However, conditions like heart disease present very differently across the population. Medical students and young doctors have regularly been taught to recognise heart disease by using classic examples – generally based on a male patient in his sixties. While the most common symptom of a heart attack is chest pain, women are more likely to experience other symptoms including breast discomfort, pain between their shoulder blades, nausea, vomiting or shortness of breath. This leads to an increased risk of heart attacks being missed in women, causing delays in appropriate treatment and less favourable long-term outcomes.[1]

This inequality also continues when it comes to managing pain. It's a tragedy that female patients presenting to the emergency department often aren't taken as seriously or treated as compassionately as male patients with the same symptoms. They wait longer before receiving treatment and are less likely to be given painkillers.[2]

This male-centric approach when it comes to medical research even translates into an increased risk of women dying in a car accident. For decades crash test dummies were built to resemble the average man, meaning their proportions and weight distribution differed dramatically from the average woman. And even then it's only been in recent years that test dummies supposed to represent women evolved beyond just a scaled-down version of the original male model. Similarly, seatbelts have not been designed in a way to protect people who are pregnant in a crash.[3]

And when it comes to studying sex, clitoral anatomy has been largely ignored in comparison to the penis. It's only recently that this important part of female genitalia has been given the attention it deserves.[4]

We've clearly got a long way to go, but fortunately the tables are starting to turn.

There is a push to recruit female participants for medical research, which will thankfully broaden our understanding of the differences in treating all sexes.

Gender-specific presentations are being studied, acknowledged and taught to the next generation of doctors. This will ultimately improve the speed and accuracy of diagnosis, as well as improve the management and health outcomes for every patient. Sensitivity to patient needs, experiences and desired health outcomes are also being emphasised in research, allowing everyone to have a voice in their own care.

On the other side of the stethoscope, we've been lucky enough to have gender parity when it comes to medical training in Australia for several decades, but the legacy of male dominion in medicine remains.

In Australia, women only represent twenty-eight per cent of medical deans and 12.5 per cent of hospital chief executive officers.[5] There's also a difference in specialty choices; where female physicians tend to pursue careers in obstetrics, gynaecology or paediatrics, other specialties like radiology and orthopaedics are still predominantly male.

For as long as women continue to encounter male-dominated, patronising or disrespectful health services, then fear and distrust of modern medical practices will remain – preventing women from receiving the medical care they desperately need.

The self-perpetuating system of male leadership in medicine has created a space where some women feel uncomfortable, and this suspicion of the medical establishment has created a gap in the market for 'wellness' to step in.

Nonsense therapies are often peddled towards women – marketed as wellness products – while also framing health concerns as lifestyle issues rather than encouraging people to seek a solution based in science.

Wellness products aimed at a female demographic may state their goal is to be sensitive to their specific needs or to empower the consumer, but they are often predatory and exploitative.

Women are bombarded with unhealthy messages from childhood to old age. Money can be made by telling people that they continually need to strive to become more beautiful, more sexy and less wrinkled.

Celebrity endorsements are very successful when it comes to selling fitness regimens, clothing, hair, makeup and recipe books. Instagram influencers promote diet products that perpetuate unattainable ideals, which only serves to increase the potential to worsen mental health and drive up disordered eating.

Female wellness products generally follow five themes: the advertising uses complex and technical science terminology, usually out of context; they prey on some women's insecurities, including body image; they claim to be 'chemical free' and natural; they claim to originate from traditional or ancient wisdom; and they provide 'spiritual healing'.

The list of wellness products, services and therapies is long and continually growing, but let's take a look at some of the notable offenders.

VAMPIRE FACIALS

This 'anti-ageing' treatment has been promoted by many celebrities including Gwyneth Paltrow and Kim Kardashian.

It, rather disgustingly, involves taking a sample of your blood and injecting it back into your face.

Blood is withdrawn from your veins, placed in a test tube and spun in a centrifuge. During this process red blood cells fall to the bottom of the tube, while the lighter plasma sits at the top. This yellow-tinged plasma is syphoned into a syringe and then injected back into your face.

It all sounds rather vampirey and gross. A similar procedure is used for sporting injuries – taking blood, spinning it down and injecting platelet-rich plasma (PRP) back into your tendons, muscles or joints. These treatments are not called 'vampire sports shots' – but they should be.

Vampire facials have the added benefit of being perfect for the Instagram age as they look impressively horrific. Celebrities and online influencers shock their followers by posting selfies of their swollen face covered in hundreds of bloodstained injection sites.

Some therapists even skip a step. By not spinning the blood in a centrifuge and just injecting it back into your face, you're left looking like an overzealous teenage vampire wearing braces has had a nibble.

These plasma injections are meant to stimulate collagen production within your skin, making it appear more plump and less wrinkled. However, the main outcome is likely to be facial swelling. 'Anti-ageing' effects disappear after a few days when the swelling subsides, which inspires some people to get regular weekly vampire facials in an attempt to maintain their vampiric youth.[6]

BEE STING FACIALS

Health treatments derived from honeybees are called apitherapy and include using honey, propolis, royal jelly and bee venom. The most hideous type of apitherapy is called a 'bee sting facial', which uses live bees to sting your face – those poor bees – and a close second is 'live bee acupuncture', which stings you everywhere else.

It's unsurprisingly painful for you, but it's much worse for the bees because after they sting you, they die.

Wrinkles appear reduced due to the bee venom swelling up your face, but the effect doesn't last long. It can also be dangerous. This is definitely not the kind of facial you should try if you are allergic to bee venom. Even if you're not allergic, there's no guarantee of safety.

In 2018, a 55-year-old woman in Spain had an adverse reaction to bee acupuncture. She had been regularly attending apitherapy sessions every month for two years with no history of problems until one session, out of the blue, she experienced an anaphylactic reaction and died.[7]

Most people go out of their way to avoid bee stings, not elect to have them take place on your face. Just because something sounds trendy and scary, doesn't mean you need to try it.

NON-TOXIC TAMPONS

Sterile, mass-produced tampons have been available for about eighty years, but recently there has been a move to ditch these clean, individually wrapped, insertable tampons and use something more natural – like a sea sponge.

We know that commercially produced sterile tampons are safe when used correctly, yet some companies encourage women to put them aside and use a sea sponge fished out of the ocean instead.

They're washed, but this does not mean they are necessarily sterile. They might be quite good at absorbing period blood, but bacteria can hide in all of their nooks and crannies. The vagina provides a moist, warm space where bacteria can thrive and proliferate into a hideous, persistent and potentially fatal vaginal infection.

The string attached to a manufactured tampon is designed to pull the tampon out completely, but natural sponges taken from the sea floor don't have strings and are much more difficult to remove. Parts of the sponge can break off and secretly remain inside the vagina, leading to toxic shock syndrome, the development of sepsis and an emergency situation.

The early signs of pelvic inflammatory disease can be similar to period pain so by the time someone thinks about seeing a doctor, it's pretty serious.

NATURAL BREAST ENLARGEMENT

Breast enlargement surgery can obviously make a dramatic difference to the size of your breasts, but some people may not want to go through an operation or can't afford it. Non-surgical therapies have popped up to offer more gentle, affordable and natural alternatives in the form of pills, massage, lotions and hypnosis. Unfortunately, none of these more conservative options works nearly as effectively as an operation.

Pills may marginally increase your breast size if they contain the female hormone oestrogen, but this prescription medication should really be used under medical supervision as it could increase your risk of breast cancer, blood clots, worsening migraines or a stroke.

Massages are sometimes advertised as the answer, and while they might temporarily enhance blood flow, they won't increase your cup size.

The most out-there treatment I've heard of is the use of hypnosis to convince your brain that you're going through puberty again. Why anybody would choose to go through puberty twice is beyond me. Hypnosis isn't known to increase your oestrogen level, but even if it did, your body wouldn't be able to selectively enhance your breast size without giving you everything else that goes along with the teenage change, including pimples and a debilitating emotional rollercoaster.

YONI EGGS

When I think about people placing jade eggs into their vagina I think of Gwyneth Paltrow. Her health and fitness company Goop targets women and sells wellness and lifestyle products to their customers. In 2017 they started promoting yoni eggs, claiming they could 'balance hormones, regulate menstrual cycles, prevent uterine prolapse, and increase bladder control'.[8]

These egg-shaped crystals were advertised to be a secret, ancient healing therapy, carefully guarded by Chinese royalty. Ultimately, they made the case that placing egg-shaped crystals inside your vagina would improve your sex life.

There was an understandable outcry from health professionals around the world, concerned these claims were misleading. Like a sea sponge, inserting a non-sterile crystal egg into your vagina could potentially introduce harmful bacteria. Leaving it in for too long could also cause toxic shock syndrome and sepsis.

An investigation found that Goop's health claims regarding the yoni eggs were not backed by scientific evidence and in September 2018, Paltrow's lifestyle brand agreed to pay a USD$145,000 fine to the Orange County District Attorney's Office.[9]

Goop withdrew their original statements about the eggs' use, but the crystals continue to be sold on their website. While they are still intended for vaginal insertion, they now claim that yoni eggs can harness the power of crystal healing and energy work – which is at least a subtle improvement.

The company has come under fire many times since, like when they sold a product called the 'Inner Judge Flower Essence Blend', a formula that could be placed on your tongue to 'help prevent depression'.[10]

Depression is a serious mental health condition that can be life threatening and needs to be carefully monitored by health professionals. It's bold to claim it can be prevented by placing flower essence drops on your tongue.

•

These therapies may seem ridiculous, but like many of the treatments discussed in this book, the marketing is designed to be manipulative. When someone has already tried and failed to lose weight, look younger or increase their breast size, a new option can seem mighty appealing.

The male-dominated medical world must also shoulder some of the blame for this. Women have not been sitting at the decision-making table for centuries. Their experiences have been discounted and this has driven many people away from seeking science-based therapies and into the arms of charlatans.

It is simply unacceptable to take advantage of people, and those in positions of power need to do better than trick consumers into buying useless products or encourage the insertion of crystals into their vaginas.

The arrival of more female doctors in our hospitals and clinics can only change medicine for the better. But at the moment a gap exists between what women expect from healthcare services and the treatment they receive. We need to create environments within medical clinics and services where women feel safe, comfortable and heard.

Similarly we need to incentivise and enable women when they are keen to pursue their medical career in a typically male-dominated specialty.

We also need to stop promoting unrealistic body expectations and stop faking before and after shots to promote health products. And we need to dismantle the systemic structures that encourage harmful attitudes about body image, especially from a young age.

CHAPTER 11

LOSING IT

One of my pet hates is seeing 'miracle weight loss pills' getting flogged online. So you can imagine my surprise when I discovered I was selling them one day.

It was a lazy Sunday morning in September 2020 – I was eating brunch outside in the sun when I received an email from an irate woman from New Zealand. Kathleen's message was straight to the point:

> Hi, I have just purchased your product and was horrified when I went into my bank account to see two lots of money taken out ... Your false advertising stated this product was much cheaper than the amount taken out of my account. I no longer want this product. Very unhappy!!!

I had no idea what she was talking about. So I did what anyone else would do – I assumed it was a scam and continued eating my porridge, until I received another email a few minutes later from Michelle in Melbourne:

Hi Brad, just checking if you actually are promoting the product called Keto Premiere, or are they using you without your consent?

I started to worry – surely there had been some mistake?

I responded to both Kathleen and Michelle and quickly realised I had a very serious problem on my hands.

Then more people started reaching out. There was no denying what was happening – someone had stolen my identity and was diddling people out of their money.

'The excess weight will disappear. 100% natural. 100% organic'

'Free Trial. How mother of 2 finally drops 3 dress sizes after being overweight for years!'

'Important information!!! Wear jeans 5 sizes smaller. Will women over 61kg be surprised?'

My trustworthy face was being used to sell diet pills.

I was shocked to see myself superimposed in front of luscious lemons and ripe raspberries, peddling pills across the Asia–Pacific region.

The advertisements were a bit dodgy with vague language, lots of spelling mistakes and empty promises, but they were authentic enough to draw people in.

It turns out Kathleen was a woman in her mid-sixties who had been targeted by advertising on Facebook and fallen for the scam. Trusting my face, she'd handed over her credit card details to buy some keto pills and before she knew it, several transactions had been taken from her account – adding up to almost five hundred dollars.

She was understandably angry.

The advertisements themselves were quite sophisticated. Clicking on the ad took unsuspecting people to a mocked-up version of a *New Zealand Herald* article, where I supposedly declared these pills would change people's lives. An imitation of an *ABC News* article soon followed. The headline was somewhat complicated, but enough to fool people: 'Australia will get 12500 packets of a universal weight loss product by the institute of nutritional science as a special price'.

They had even given me a new biography: 'Leading Australian nutritionist, holder of a Habilitation degree in Medicine at the Institute of Nutritional Science, Australia, professor, developer of a weight loss method, author of books about weight loss, a well known TV & radio host. Work experience: 42 years. The most famous people not only from Australia, but also from all over the world entrust their body shape and health to him.'

I was outraged – primarily because I am not yet forty-two years old, let alone having forty-two years of work experience under my belt. I couldn't let this deceitful lie about my age go unchallenged, something had to be done!

Of course, the rest of the résumé was a fabricated word salad too.

I posted warnings on my social media accounts, asked my followers to be careful, alerted the ABC, called my medical indemnity team and contacted Scamwatch.

Scamwatch is an offshoot of the Australian Competition and Consumer Commission (ACCC) and according to its website, it 'provides information to consumers and small businesses about how to recognise, avoid and report scams'.

I went to their web page to report the problem and ask for help, but then I noticed their disclaimer: 'The ACCC is unable to help you recover money lost to a scam or assist in tracking down a scammer.'[1]

I had assumed this organisation would be like the Scooby gang – solving crimes and tracking down fraudsters – but 'Scamwatch' was more appropriately named than I expected. They only watch scams.

The ABC's investigative team tracked my identity thieves to Ukraine but then the trail went cold.[2]

Unfortunately, I discovered that when someone steals your identity and uses it to sell weight loss products, there is very little you can do.

It's the ultimate betrayal, seeing your own face selling the very thing you despise. I went through a bizarre range of emotions, but my own annoyance and irritation was nothing compared to the anxiety and anger felt by the people who emailed me – lovely people who had seen the ads pop up on Facebook and innocently clicked to buy weight loss pills from what appeared to be a trustworthy source – me!

Targeted ad campaigns can be effective because they appeal to our vulnerabilities. You might be keen to lose weight, but too embarrassed to speak with your doctor about it – a quick weight loss solution in the form of a bottle of pills might seem like the answer, but even without the scams it's a risky business.

•

Diet trends and weight loss products go in and out of fashion. Currently, one of the more popular fads is the ketogenic diet – eating a high amount of protein and fat, but a very low amount of carbohydrates. Meals consist of lean meat, eggs, cheese, fish, nuts, butter, oils, seeds and some vegetables. Carbohydrate-loaded root vegetables including potatoes, sweet potatoes, carrots and parsnips are off the list.

The diet also advises against whole grains, pasta, cereals, rice, beans and legumes. Processed food and anything containing sugar is off limits too. This includes lollies, smoothies, cake, cow's milk, ice-cream, fruit juice and fruit. You're not about to drink alcohol any time soon either.

Keto is based on a simple metabolic principle – our cells prefer a steady intake of carbohydrates to work efficiently, but if carbohydrates aren't readily available in our bloodstream, we've got a separate metabolic pathway (like a backup generator) that still allows our body to function – a process called ketosis.

Your body breaks down fat to produce ketones which it uses as an alternative energy source. Fat cells decrease in size as the energy contained within them is released and you start losing weight.

It's common to experience aching muscles and feel lethargic after commencing keto. This sensation is affectionately referred to as 'keto flu' but usually disappears after a few days when your body reaches its 'new normal'.

Side effects include bad breath, abdominal cramps, constipation, nausea, vomiting and sometimes insomnia. This can make keto an unpleasant experience for people following the diet, as well as their household contacts.

It's common to lose weight after starting keto, particularly if you were eating a lot of junk food before taking it up. But the diet is difficult to follow over a long period of time and many people soon give up and go back to their old ways.

Weight that is lost from following any diet is difficult to keep off, and it's no different with keto.

That's a basic introduction to the keto world, and the pills my face were selling are meant to help this process take place.

But keto pills are different from the keto diet. They are advertised as a weight loss solution, but the reasoning behind them is flawed.

I asked accredited dietitian Linda Cumines what was in keto pills and if they worked. She told me they contain 'Beta-hydroxybutyrate, which is a ketone body in its own right.' She continued, 'It doesn't actually make sense. How can adding ketones make you burn fat even more? It's your body that's got to produce the ketones to reduce weight.'

Instead of breaking down your own fat stores in order to lose weight, your body uses the keto pills as its energy source and leaves your stored fat exactly where it is.[3]

As a gentle reminder, weight loss pill scammers don't care about your health. Their primary goal is to take your money.

●

Mandy-Lee Noble is an accredited dietitian in Brisbane who has been researching diets for years. When asked if fad diets or diet pills are successful, she doesn't beat around the bush: 'No diet has evidence of providing significant weight loss in the majority of people long term (two to five years). Essentially no diets are helpful.'

It might feel deflating to hear this from a dietitian, but Mandy-Lee said it's not our fault, 'Human bodies are biologically "hard wired" to defend their highest adult body weight. Any sort of calorie restriction is met by the mechanisms of body weight homeostasis.'

This means that your body is constantly trying to conserve energy and no matter how long you might diet, it always tries to return to its highest set point.

No wonder it's so difficult to lose weight and even harder to keep it off. Losing weight takes time and effort. Keeping it off requires permanent lifestyle change. So why do people keep spending money on quick-fix solutions?

Mandy-Lee told me it wasn't clear cut, 'I think the answer to that is very complex. I don't have a lived experience of being in a larger body, but I can tell you, from working primarily with clients that do, that they mostly want to desperately get out from underneath the relentless suffering of weight stigma.

'People in bigger bodies are under constant attack from a socially accepted form of discrimination, and people in smaller and middle-size bodies are aware of this – and terrified of it,' she said. 'Weight loss and all of its associated scams thrive due to how people are treated.'

Buying weight loss products and diet books from the anonymous comfort of your own home is far less confronting than subjecting yourself to possible ridicule or embarrassment at a medical clinic.

We know it's hard to lose weight. We've all been told before that we need to eat less and move more, but the promise of rapid weight loss by simply taking tablets is appealing.

However, purchasing pills online is like buying recreational drugs at a bus stop – you could have the best time of your life or you could wind up in hospital needing a new liver. It's risky, but many people are willing to take that risk.

There is little, if any, regulation for many of the weight loss pills sold online, especially from scammers, so you never know what you're going to get.

In January 2016, *The Medical Journal of Australia* published a case study of a 26-year-old man from Western Australia who presented to hospital after experiencing six weeks of fatigue. He was previously healthy and didn't smoke cigarettes, drink excessive amounts of alcohol or take recreational drugs.[4]

His initial blood tests showed he had severe liver damage, but his doctors weren't able to work out what had caused it. The medical team spoke with him further and discovered that ten weeks earlier he had started taking two dietary supplements – protein powder with a high concentration of green tea extract and a weight loss supplement containing garcinia cambogia. He took them for a week, but stopped taking both of them after getting the shivers.

Two months after presenting to hospital, he received a liver transplant that saved his life.

In February 2016, Matthew Whitby decided to go public with his story and warned others about the potential dangers of weight loss products. At the end of the day, we may never know the exact cause of his liver failure, but the green tea extract was thought to be the most likely culprit.[5]

•

Processed and pre-packaged foods are often irresistibly delicious, but they will frequently contain added sugar and hidden calories that are purposefully put in there to hit our sweet spot. In fact, scientists have a term for it: the 'bliss point'.

This is the exact point when food has the right mixture of salt, sugar and fat to maximise the delicious nature of the item you're eating. American market researcher and food scientist Howard Moskowitz describes the bliss point as 'that sensory profile where you like food the most'.[6]

Food companies use the bliss point to make their products more enticing and keep us coming back for more.

We're set up to fail!

These days, calories are cheap and it's easy to gain weight. All of us have the propensity to put weight on, particularly as we get older. This is a global issue, and we are seeing entire populations become overweight, even in developing countries where food was once scarce.

And it's not just our food making us gain weight. Prescribed medication can increase our appetite and slow down metabolism, while mental health problems like stress, anxiety and depression can drive us towards comfort food and prevent us from feeling like exercising. Physical injuries limit our movement and can make exercise difficult or impossible. Even being overweight will decrease our ability to exercise, so it can be a vicious cycle.

One in five Australian adults were obese in the mid-1990s, and that number has continued to increase – in 2018, it was one in three.[7]

No wonder a significant proportion of the population turn to dieting to lose weight.

Fad diets seem pervasive. Everyone knows about them and ads for them are everywhere. So how do we know which ones to choose? And, more importantly, do any of them work?

Popular diets are designed to lure people in with all kinds of exotic vegetables, 'superfoods' and timed eating rituals, but Mandy-Lee stressed that it's important to remember their aim is not to make us healthier. Fad diets are not a long-term plan for sustained health, but a shorter-term tool for rapid weight loss. People diet to lose weight and fad diets are a response to the societal pressure to look thin.

She told me there was no way to keep track of all the fad diets currently on offer, 'there really is an endless list and they evolve and shapeshift over time'.

But there are plenty of similarities between them, so Mandy-Lee recommends boiling them down to the actual mechanism of weight loss, even if the weight loss is only short-lived.

They can generally be placed into three categories: restrictive, elimination and ideological diets.

RESTRICTIVE DIETS

Restrictive diets approach eating with limitations, either by placing a daily limit on the hours you're able to eat, the total number of calories you can eat over the day, or both. In some restrictive diets, you're able to consume whatever you like but need to stop eating once you've reached your daily calorie limit.

The best example of this is intermittent fasting.

Intermittent fasting

Modern eating habits typically include three meals a day plus additional snacks when we're feeling peckish. Easy access to the pantry and local supermarket means we rarely run out of food and our body gets a steady supply of nutrition. Intermittent fasting is a different approach to eating, which includes periods of little or no calorie intake.

It regularly forces your body into starvation mode. The energy stored in your fat is mobilised and you lose weight. Intermittent fasting gets your body used to breaking down fat stores more readily and encourages this metabolic pathway to be more active.

The 5:2 diet, popularised by Dr Michael Mosley, encourages you to eat a moderate amount of food on five days of the week, and a smaller amount on the other two days.

Another way to fast intermittently is to split each day into two parts – eating and non-eating.

The 16:8 eating program allocates eight hours each day where you can eat, and the remaining sixteen hours are for fasting.

Restrictive diets also include 'alternate day fasting', 'eat stop eat', and 'the warrior diet'. These all have restrictions on the times of the day or on which days of the week you're allowed to eat.

My friend Vincent became obsessed with intermittent fasting. He followed the 5:2 diet but it didn't work for him. He moved to the 16:8 diet, and then the 18:6. He finally pushed himself to try out the 20:4 diet but fainted.

ELIMINATION DIETS

Elimination diets focus on excluding – or extremely limiting – particular foods or food groups. A classic example of this is the Atkins Diet.

Atkins Diet

Dr Robert Atkins was a cardiologist who released his book *Dr Atkins' Diet Revolution* in 1972. It was a bestseller and helped popularise his eating program, appropriately and proudly named the 'Atkins Diet'.

His book recommended consuming a low-carbohydrate and high-fat diet, which flew in the face of the popular understanding of food at the time. It was commonly thought that eating fatty food made you put on weight, so all you needed to do was eat lean meat and cut the fat off your bacon and you'd be right. So it was understandably shocking that some proponents of the Atkins Diet even suggested that you can eat all the fat you want and still lose weight, provided you keep your carbohydrates to a minimum.

It's still a popular diet today and many people swear by it, noticing rapid weight loss, especially in the first few weeks. But initial weight loss is common in many diets, mainly due to losing fluid and muscle mass rather than reducing fat.

Quick weight loss is a good start, but what matters more is sustaining it long term. Previous research showed people were able to lose weight after six months but had a tendency to return to their original weight after twelve months. They also found the diet was difficult to maintain over the long term.[8]

However, a recent evaluation of popular diets in 2017 actually showed the Atkins Diet could be beneficial for maintaining weight loss even at twelve months, so the jury is still out.[9]

Throughout the 1960s and 1970s, fat was demonised while low-fat and fat-free products started appearing on the shelves.

We're now facing an obesity crisis around the world and it's easy to look back and recognise something clearly went wrong a few decades ago. The reasons for this predicament are complex, but one likely cause is this alteration in our diet.

Foods that are low in fat have a tendency to be unsatisfying and can result in us consuming more calories to feel full. Low-fat foods are also often unpalatable, so the sugar content is cranked up to compensate. This might hit your bliss point, but lots of sugar isn't exactly healthy for you, and often contributes to weight gain.

In 1965, a literature review of coronary heart disease was published in the *New England Journal of Medicine* pointing the finger directly at fatty food as the major cause of heart disease. The review had been sponsored by the Sugar Research Foundation but this relationship was not disclosed at the time.

In November 2016, a study was published that highlighted communication within the sugar industry, showing how they were purposefully pulling the strings behind the scenes to create an image that fat was bad and sugar wasn't anything to worry about.[10]

The effect on our food industry has been long-standing and in our supermarkets we're still surrounded by products proudly displaying their fat-free status, while secretly harbouring high amounts of sucrose.

Putting this all into perspective, the Atkins Diet was a rather bold move at the time. Dr Atkins bucked the trend and took on the sugar industry with his contrary ideas. He made people less afraid of fat and more concerned about sugar, but overall, healthy eating lies somewhere in the middle. Both sides need to be factored into the equation.

So, let's look at the flip side of the coin – going sugar-free.

I Quit Sugar

As too much sugar in your diet increases your risk of gaining weight, high blood pressure, diabetes, fatty liver disease, tooth decay, heart disease and stroke, it's a good idea to limit it. But in 2018 nearly fifty per cent of Australians consumed too much of the sweet stuff.[11]

For many people, reducing sugar means only having one teaspoon in your tea instead of two. This is a good start, but it's only the tip of the iceberg because there's so much extra sugar hidden in all of our foods.[12]

I Quit Sugar started out as a blog by Sarah Wilson in 2011, encouraging readers to eliminate refined sugar from their diets. Over time it evolved into a company with a range of cookbooks, detox programs and more. Sarah motivated her followers to check their foods for all forms of sugar – white, brown, palm and coconut sugar, as well as avoiding lollies, chocolate, jams, tomato sauces, honey, agave, flavoured yoghurt and fruit.

Soft drinks were also discouraged – a single can may contain up to ten teaspoons of the stuff. The World Health Organization (WHO) recommends people consume fewer than six teaspoons each day so a single can of soft drink could take you over the limit.

Sarah was not qualified as a dietitian or nutritionist, but used her own experience and research to teach others how to eat. Despite her best intentions, the diet was criticised for recommending foods that still contained hidden sugars – like organic rice malt syrup. It contains fifty-four per cent sugar – just in a slightly different form.

Dietitians like Mandy-Lee noticed that when Sarah shared her dietary advice with the world, 'she was merely swapping one sugar with another'.

'I am often reminding people that your body does not care about the provenance of the glucose transiting through your digestive tract.'

Overall, cutting down on sugar is a magnificent aspiration and should be commended, but replacing it with other forms that are metabolised in a similar way defeats the purpose.

Sarah Wilson dissolved her relationship with *I Quit Sugar* in 2018.

IDEOLOGICAL DIETS

Ideological diets are based on an idea, theory or ethical framework, but not necessarily on science or common sense. This includes vegetarian diets where people choose to abstain from eating meat, vegan diets where all animal products are out, and raw food diets where food is eaten as it comes without being cooked. But apart from these, my favourite example is the Palaeolithic diet.

Paleo Diet

The Paleo diet was popularised in Australia by former celebrity chef, Pete Evans, but it has been around for the past few decades. In 2002, health scientist Loren Cordain published his book *The Paleo Diet*, which sparked an interest around the world in this way of eating.

It's often marketed as a caveman diet and is based on the theory that humans evolved in tandem with the food available to our hunter–gatherer Palaeolithic ancestors. It's thought that as we've introduced modern agricultural practices and entered into the industrial age, we've moved away from the food sources that perfectly complement our bodies, and this is why humans have collectively become more unhealthy and overweight over time.

But the entire premise of this diet is shrouded in doubt for many reasons.

To begin with, it just doesn't make sense.

The Palaeolithic era spans from roughly 2.5 million years ago until about ten thousand years ago, and during this time our Paleo ancestors lived all over the globe and ate a wide variety of food.

Paleo is a high-protein and low-carbohydrate diet, with lean meat and plenty of fresh vegetables. Foods produced through modern agricultural processes and technology are out, including wheat, cereals, whole grains, legumes, beans, cow's milk and processed foods. However, choosing to exclude these from your diet can contribute to problems later in life.

The life expectancy of our Palaeolithic ancestors was much younger than what we expect today, so the Paleo diet may not provide adequate nutrition for an elderly population.

Osteoporosis is more likely to occur as you get older, where calcium is slowly whittled away from inside your bones, making them prone to fractures. It's important to have a steady supply of calcium in your diet to prevent osteoporosis from happening. We usually recommend including regular serves of cow's milk, yoghurt and cheese in your diet as these are all rich sources of calcium, but these foods are excluded in the Paleo diet.

Whole grains are known to reduce the risk of bowel cancer but are not included in Paleo.

On the positive side, plenty of people love Paleo. They've ditched processed food and started using fresh ingredients. They're excited about cooking again and making wiser food choices. Some have lost weight and even gotten rid of their diabetes. They'll just need to monitor carefully in the future for osteoporosis and bowel cancer.

HERE'S A HANDY GUIDE TO
TRANSLATING FAD DIET JARGON

'Rapid weight loss.' = 'You'll rapidly become dehydrated.'

'You'll never believe these results.' = 'Don't believe these results.'

'This study shows ...' = 'We've finally found a study that shows ...'

'Doctors won't tell you ...' = 'Doctors already know this doesn't work.'

'Stimulates natural weight loss.' = 'Please believe our product is natural.'

'This book holds the key.' = 'I get a cut of the sales.'

'One hundred per cent of people are satisfied.' = 'No one is satisfied.'

'Elimination diet.' = 'You may become vitamin deficient.'

'Karen lost ten kilos in ten days.' = 'Science says it doesn't work, but please believe Karen.'

NOT-SO-FAD DIETS

Compared to the fashionable diets that come and go, some diets have a bit more staying power. Following are just two examples of medically recommended diets.

Mediterranean Diet

One of the most fondly favoured diets in medical circles is the Mediterranean. It's primarily recommended as a way of eating to help you live longer, but there is also evidence that it reduces the risk of developing diabetes, heart disease, dementia, some cancers and can help maintain a healthy weight.

This plant-based diet encourages the consumption of fresh vegetables, legumes, fruit, whole grains, nuts and herbs. It's also okay to eat small amounts of lean meat, chicken, eggs and the occasional serve of Greek yoghurt. You can also enjoy seafood, fish and olive oil, which contain omega-3 fats that may help improve your cholesterol.

Processed food is off the menu, but Mediterranean food is fortunately rather tasty.

Dairy products are minimal, so it's important to keep an eye on your calcium intake and increase it if necessary.

There are lots of healthy options and the Mediterranean diet can be great for communal eating and bringing the family together (when you're not in a pandemic).

DASH Diet

This is healthy eating for medical nerds. DASH stands for Dietary Approaches to Stop Hypertension, and it's an eating plan developed by the National Heart, Lung and Blood Institute in the US. This diet originally spawned from observing that people who ate a mostly plant-based diet were less likely to develop high blood pressure.

It focuses on eating fresh vegetables, fruit, whole grains, lean meats, nuts, seeds and legumes. It's low in salt, red meat, sugary foods and fat, but doesn't eliminate them completely.

The diet is also known to reduce weight, help prevent metabolic syndrome, decrease the chance of type 2 diabetes, and may also reduce the risk of developing some cancers, including colorectal and breast cancer.

The DASH diet might be familiar if you work in health care, but otherwise it's not extremely popular in Australia.

This diet is well balanced and has plenty of variety, so you're less likely to suffer any particular nutritional deficits.

●

The Dietitians Association of Australia found that nearly half (forty-six per cent) of Australian adults surveyed in 2017 had tried to lose weight in the previous year, and nearly half (forty-seven per cent) of these people had spent money on a specific diet or diet program.[13] This means that about a quarter of the Australian adult population are spending money on weight loss products or diets. That's a lot of people spending a lot of money.

It's best not to gain the extra pounds in the first place, but what can you do if it's already happened? Basic advice is to exercise regularly, eat a wide variety of vegetables, and don't eat too much.

Of course, other factors include your past medical history, medication, metabolism, income, genetics, environment, exercise, your general relationship with food and how motivated you are. But there are no miracle solutions for weight loss. It's not just knowing how to eat or how to exercise, it's having the motivation to do it.

Guidance from a dietitian or exercise physiologist can help monitor your weight and fitness level, hold you accountable, offer a professional perspective and provide you with evidence-based information. This is a much better approach than trying to do it on your own and you're more likely to be successful with weight reduction over the longer term if you slowly, steadily and consistently chip away at it.

And if you see my face selling natural weight loss pills, it's pretty safe to conclude my identity has been stolen again.

CHAPTER 12

DETOXES AND CLEANSES

Frivolous living and debaucherous behaviour can leave party animals feeling tired, stressed out or hungover. Fun nights are often followed by terrible days of headaches, nausea, dry mouth, bad breath, muscle cramps, high anxiety and worsening depression. Flashbacks from the night before can make us shudder in regret while we're curled up in the fetal position crying.

It's not just those messy nights out, even fabulous holidays full of fine friends and fine dining can leave us bloated and a few kilograms heavier.

In these times of despair and disappointment we'll typically reach out for anything that might be an instant fix. Detoxes and cleanses fill this niche in the market and are promoted as the fastest way to get your body back into shape and feeling normal – but it's all just a commercial ploy.

A friend of mine, Brendan, was in the best shape of his life before his wedding day. Hours at the gym had been worth it and paying close attention to his diet had worked. Twelve months later everything had changed. He realised he had been drinking too much alcohol, eating too much food and not exercising. Meanwhile, married life had been treating his wife well as she had been eating healthy food, training every day and competing in triathlons.

She inspired him to do something about it and he informed me that he was starting his health kick with a 'liver detox cleanse'.

He would only eat fresh vegetables, say goodbye to alcohol and had bought some liver detox tablets from the local pharmacy. He had no idea what was in them or what toxins would be purged from his liver, only that they were sure to make him lose weight. He had just grabbed them off the shelf.

Your liver generally doesn't need additional help from pills – it rejuvenates itself when given the chance. I suggested to Brendan that eating vegetables and stopping the booze would do all the work, while the liver cleansing tablets were just a distraction – but he wasn't convinced. The power of marketing had told him that these tablets were essential to starting his new life.

Medical doctors will talk about 'detoxing' our patients if they have had an overdose or they need help withdrawing from alcohol or other addictive drugs. But the word 'detox' has been hijacked, twisted into a marketing gimmick to help move products off the shelves.

My first experience witnessing a detox in action felt like I had stepped into a scene from *The Exorcist*. As a medical student, I diligently turned up to the emergency department early in the morning to join the doctors' handover meeting. The team gathered near the main desk to talk about the patients, and just opposite us was a teenage girl sitting on the side of her bed, dressed in a crisp white hospital gown.

The emergency consultant from the night shift yawned his way through the whiteboard of patient names, and as he told us about Cindy he motioned to the young girl.

She had been brought into hospital after taking an unknown quantity of alcohol and tablets, and now a nasogastric tube had been stuck up her nose and it went all the way down into her stomach. It had been used to suck up as much fluid from her gut as possible, then liquid charcoal was pumped back down the tube in an attempt to soak up anything remaining.

Cindy started to groan, and as she turned to face us, I couldn't help but notice the black liquid dripping down the front of her gown. She opened her mouth, revealing charcoal-stained teeth, before projectile vomiting like a garden sprinkler spurting oil.

This is the image I think of when I think of a detox.

Detoxification might be a great solution after your neighbour has invited you over for a cup of English breakfast tea and laced it with arsenic, or if you're a member of Russia's opposition party.

It can be lifesaving in certain situations, but detoxification isn't helpful when the problem is that you've been eating too many cheeseburgers.

Patients may need to be admitted to hospital for a detox when they have been regularly drinking too much alcohol, snorting methamphetamine or injecting heroin. Suddenly ceasing these substances can lead to an uncomfortable withdrawal syndrome, with sensations like nausea, vomiting, muscle pain and abdominal cramps. It can also cause more serious health concerns like confusion, delirium, collapse, coma, seizures or death.

But I frequently see patients who have been hitting the sauce a little too hard over summer who decide to go on a month of 'detoxing' to give their body a break. They stop drinking alcohol, eat more vegetables, decrease red meat, flood themselves with water, and if they are really into it, they'll start taking a liver detox supplement. When they make these significant changes to their lifestyle, they begin to feel better. They report feeling more clear-headed, having more energy and fewer muscular aches and pains. They attribute this improved feeling of wellbeing to their detox supplement, but don't realise that it's just because they are taking care of themselves and are not perpetually hungover.

The promise of a detox is pretty close to religious redemption. You're told that you can imbibe on the weekend with copious amounts of alcohol, junk food, recreational drugs and no sleep – just make sure you consume a large green detox smoothie in the morning to ameliorate all your previous indiscretions.

The modern marketing concept behind a detox is to suggest that toxins continually accumulate in our bodies and will cause us harm unless we use a detox to get rid of them.

However, these 'toxins' are never specifically named, making it impossible to determine if a detox has actually made an impact.

Pills, potions, tinctures and tonics claim to detox your liver, but the truth is that with time and a healthy diet your body will detox itself. Your internal organs have evolved to do this without special products from the health food shop.

It can't be denied that some people do feel better after using detox products. This can often be due to the placebo effect, where we make a conscious choice to improve our health and convince ourselves we're feeling better. But detox pills, juices and teas can have some harmful effects.

Many of them contain diuretics and laxatives.

Diuretics encourage your kidneys to make more urine. You'll temporarily lose weight because you're dehydrated, but this fluid will return soon after you stop taking the diuretic and if you don't change your lifestyle and continue eating the same food, you'll quickly end up back where you started. Laxatives work by making your stools soft or by stimulating the muscles in your intestinal wall, causing them to speed up the excretion process. This will make you go to the toilet more frequently, clearing out your bowel. This can make you feel lighter, reduce bloating and you'll even notice a difference on the bathroom scales. Detox products with laxatives might claim to rid your body of toxins, but it's not really toxins, is it? It's diarrhoea.

Will it provide you with a feeling of wellbeing and alertness? Well, yes. You'll feel accomplished after your champion bowel actions, that's for sure. You'll also be more vigilant, always alert to the location of the next bathroom.

Regular use of bowel stimulants can cause the muscles within your intestinal wall to become sluggish without them. Constipation sets in after you've stopped the bowel stimulants which leads to a cycle of dependence. This can eventually cause your bowel to become inactive and floppy, until you finally end up in the emergency department having your rectum cleared out by a young intern with a long-handled teaspoon.

So, what kinds of detoxes are out there?

LEMON DETOX DIET

There are thousands of products out there, but one of the classics of the genre is the lemon detox diet. It was originally designed as an alternative cure for stomach ulcers by American naturopath Stanley Burroughs in the 1940s before being reinvented and republished in 1976 as *The Master Cleanser*.

This detox involves replacing solid food with about eight glasses of a special lemon mixture containing water, lemon juice, cayenne pepper and tree syrup (a combination of palm syrup and maple syrup) every day, for seven to fourteen days. You're also encouraged to drink salty water, which acts as a laxative, and senna tea, a bowel stimulant.

There's nothing special about cayenne pepper, tree syrup or even lemons, but limiting your food intake and increasing your diarrhoea output will certainly cause you to temporarily lose weight.

COLONIC IRRIGATION

My good friend Deborah was a little embarrassed to tell me about her trip to the colonic irrigation clinic. She was keen to tell me about her visit because she thought it was an amazing experience – but she also knew I'd be horrified.

She'd been feeling bloated and trying to lose weight without success, so a bowel cleanse seemed like the perfect plan to help her reset and refresh her gut.

At the clinic, she stripped off her clothes and lay down on her side, while a polite practitioner took a lubricated hose attachment, aimed it at her anus and inserted it into her rectum. They filled her colon with water and then siphoned the fluid out again through a clear plastic pipe positioned in plain sight.

As her very own fecal fluid floated in front of her face, the practitioner took great delight in telling her that some of the stools flying by had been sitting inside her gut for years. She was told that having a colonic irrigation was the only way she would ever flush them out.

But your intestines are basically a very long tube. It's like a conveyor belt – what goes in one end comes out the other. I explained to Deborah that stools don't hang out in little tea rooms and coffee shops along the way before eventually feeling ready to move on.

She laughed and told me 'the proof is in the pudding'. She felt slimmer and had lost a significant amount of weight in a short amount of time, so she was happy. I told her that of course she felt slimmer and was physically lighter – the contents of her bowel had been emptied. I also explained that after a few meals she would go back to her original state, and I was right.

Colonic irrigations are a party trick to temporarily deflate your abdomen and bring down the number on the scales, but you're not losing fat – you're losing poo. They don't improve your health and can even be dangerous. Shoving fluid up your backside, especially under pressure, can cause your bowel to spring a leak. Fecal fluid then escapes your colon and ends up in your peritoneal cavity, the space surrounding your bowel and internal organs. Emergency surgery is generally needed to clear out the bacteria-laced fluid sitting around the abdomen.

Feces can also get flushed into your bloodstream which can cause an overwhelming infection. This requires plenty of intravenous antibiotics and a lengthy stay in hospital.

Thankfully my friend was all right, though disappointed – but many others have not gotten off so lightly.

CHELATION THERAPY

Chelation therapy is another type of detox used in very specific medical circumstances to remove toxic heavy metals from the body, for example when someone has been poisoned by large doses of mercury or lead.

Chemicals known as chelates are given as tablets or through intravenous infusions. They bind with heavy metals, neutralise them and carry them safely out of the body through the kidneys.

Alzheimer's disease, heart disease and autistic spectrum disorder were all once thought to be caused by heavy metal toxicity. Chelation therapy was given by health professionals as treatment, but as these conditions were found to not be caused by heavy metal toxicity, chelation has been dismally unsuccessful.

EAR CANDLING

In our quest to cleanse our bodies of gross things, we can't leave ear wax out of the conversation.

Most of us don't even think about it, but some people need their ears syringed every few months by their family doctor. Others with tricky ear canals need to see a specialist to remove their ear wax with a tiny vacuum cleaner.

It can be inconvenient, expensive or embarrassing to see your doctor about ear wax, so some people prefer home remedies they can do themselves. Ear candles would be a great treatment option, if they worked. They are frequently mistaken as credible health products, but ear candling doesn't remove ear wax and could actually cause serious harm.

Ear candles are long, hollow tubes made of wax, designed to be placed in your ear while you lay on your side. The base is positioned over the entrance of your ear canal and then the top end is lit.

You're asked to lay still while the burning candle supposedly creates a vacuum strong enough to suck out your ear wax.

After the candling session you're encouraged to grab a pair of scissors and cut down the wall of the hollow tube to reveal the contents. You'll see little lumps of wax on the inside, but they're not from your ear – it's just wax from the burning candle.

My patients don't believe me when I tell them it's just a party trick, but a simple experiment will prove it. Just light the candle when it's not sitting in your ear and you'll still see the same wax build-up within the candle.

Ear candles are not only useless, but hot wax can cause burn injuries by dripping onto your face or even into your ear canal. These products don't belong on the shelves of pharmacies.

Every now and then I'll look in a patient's ear canal and find a light layer of soot – a clear sign they've been conned.

●

We are sold the idea that our organs, bowels and ears need help to perform their daily routine – cleanses, flushes, detoxes and evacuations are all marketed on the premise that our body is unable to do its job.

But this isn't true.

Without even thinking about it, our bodies are taking care of themselves – for the most part we just need to trust our bodies and enjoy the ride.

CHAPTER 13

ANTI-VAXXERS

One morning at the clinic, a new patient attended for a medical consultation neatly dressed in a suit and tie. He was very polite and had only come to visit me for one thing: he needed me to sign a letter so his children could go to school.

It sounded like a simple request, until I asked for more information. He explained his children weren't vaccinated and he needed them to have an exemption as it was a requirement of the education department.

The request caught me off guard because he had never attended the clinic before and neither had his kids.

I asked why his children weren't immunised. Were they immunocompromised? Were they going through chemotherapy? Had they previously experienced anaphylaxis from a vaccine? If the answer was yes to any of the above, then surely the children's own doctor – someone who knew their history – should have been making these arrangements.

But no. None of these situations applied.

It's important for children to be vaccinated so that they have the opportunity to become adults. Immunisations are one of the most important health measures we can take to protect our kids and community against potentially fatal infections. Deciding not to immunise his children would not only put them at risk but would put their close contacts and the wider community at risk of infection too.

The National Immunisation Program is a schedule designed to give vaccines and booster doses at the most appropriate times of life. Some immunisations can only be given once a child's immune system has matured to a certain age, otherwise they won't work. Parents are encouraged to follow the immunisation schedule and regularly ensure their kids are up to date.

In 2015, the No Jab No Pay policy (a name that would only work in this end of the world) was brought into effect. This policy withholds government payments from families if their children are not fully immunised – essentially creating a monetary incentive for otherwise unmotivated parents and this has significantly increased vaccination rates.

The name is a spin-off from the hugely successful No Hat No Play campaign that teaches kids to wear hats when they play in the sun. The similarly named No Jab No Play policy was rolled out across Australia from 2017, requiring all children to be up to date with their immunisations in order to be enrolled in child care or school.

Parents were previously able to sign conscientious objection forms, but as immunisation affects the whole community, the Australian Government decided this was no longer a valid option.

This father was wanting a letter so his children could remain unvaccinated but still attend school, and so his family could continue receiving government benefits. I asked why he was choosing to go down this path, and he responded, 'It's because of religion. I don't want my kids to be immunised because of my religion.'

Which I knew could not be true.

Australian health authorities had already come to the conclusion that no official religion was opposed to vaccines, but this hasn't stopped many people from attempting to make such a claim over the years.[1]

In fact, the Church of Conscious Living was founded by members of an Australian anti-vaccination group with this express purpose. It wasn't successful.[2]

It eventually became apparent that my patient's usual doctor wasn't willing to sign his exemption letter, and he had been roaming the city searching for a GP who would.

He was obviously a very caring parent, wanting to protect his children from harm, but his concern was misplaced. There is overwhelming scientific evidence that vaccination is safe and effective.

It is not an easy task to convince someone who is strongly opposed to vaccines that everything is going to be okay. In fact, if done incorrectly it can backfire and help galvanise their beliefs against immunisations. This is something Associate Professor Julie Leask, a public health researcher at the University of Sydney, knows well from her studies of social responses and attitudes to vaccinations.

I asked Julie what can be done in situations like this unusual consultation, and she acknowledged that they can be difficult to manage.

She said parents fall into three different categories when it comes to this issue, 'One is where the parents are ready to vaccinate. The next is where they're very hesitant. And the third is where they're what we call declining – they're dead set not going to do it.'

For those in the third category, she advised, 'You're just not going to get anywhere, and you don't want to waste your time. You want to actually save your time for the parents who are on the fence, and who are worth investing the time in.'

For those in the middle Julie suggests more information is key to helping them make good decisions. Perhaps providing a pamphlet for them to read at their own leisure, or a link to some reputable sources.

Unfortunately, for some people vaccination is a polarising topic that can cause unnecessary conflict between friends and within families. Of course, we should all be free to make our own choices when it comes to our family's health. But this is a complicated mess when your decision not to immunise your family could harm someone else's.

●

It might seem obvious, but bacteria and viruses find their way into your body through different entry points, like your mouth, nose, throat, lungs, eyes and breaches in your skin.

Once inside it's up to your immune system to identify the new threat and respond accordingly.

One method for preventing viruses or bacteria from becoming harmful is to stop them from getting inside our bodies in the first place. This is why in the late nineteenth century the introduction of regular handwashing and widespread use of antiseptic in hospitals was extremely successful in improving public health.

More recently, during the COVID-19 pandemic, it's been drummed into us that we need to physically distance from one another, wash our hands frequently, wear face coverings and, in more extreme cases, go into lockdown.

If these measures don't work and an intruding germ enters your body, the immune system is triggered, white blood cells are mobilised, and you can get sick while they fight it off. However, your body will take steps to learn from the experience. White blood cells confront the new infection and take samples of the protein structures that line the invader's surface. The structure of these foreign proteins is then thoroughly examined by your immune system and antibodies are created to fight them. These antibodies are then pumped throughout your body, tagging the virus or bacteria that needs to be destroyed. Other cells in your immune system are then able to latch on to these antibodies, knowing they have identified the right culprit – and then they destroy it.

This process not only allows you to fight off the infection now but gives your immune system the ability to fight it off quickly in the future.

Immunisations are basically a way of showing these particular proteins to your immune system ahead of time and training your immune cells so they know what to do when the real enemy attacks. They allow your body to stop an infection in its tracks, rather than letting it wreak havoc while your immune system plays catch-up.

At the end of the day, prevention is better than cure.

The invention of vaccines has been one of the most incredible advances in human history. Yet despite extensive trials conducted in many countries around the world that continue to show vaccines are safe and effective, some people still decide not to vaccinate.

Measles is a largely preventable infection because we have an available vaccination for it, but in the first three months of 2019, the WHO recorded a massive three hundred per cent increase in people infected by measles around the world.[3]

In the final months of the same year, our Pacific neighbour, Samoa, recorded over five thousand people infected, causing an epidemic that shut down the country and left more than eighty people dead.

So how do events like this occur? And why?

●

Samoa has administered measles vaccines to their people since 1982, and prior to 2018 their childhood immunisation rates were over ninety per cent. This is good, but it's not great.

The medical community likes to reach immunisation rates over ninety-five per cent to achieve herd immunity, which means that enough people in the community are vaccinated against measles so any clusters of infection can be well contained. But in 2018, instead of improving the picturesque Polynesian island's vaccination rates even further, an unforeseen event caused them to tumble.

In July 2018, two Samoan nurses prepared MR (measles and rubella) vaccines for two one-year-old children at a medical clinic. Immunisations often come in ready-made syringes, but they're sometimes transported in a powdered form that needs to be mixed with sterile water before injecting.

Instead of mixing the powder with water, the nurses accidentally dissolved it in muscle relaxant before administering it to the two children. Soon after the immunisations were given, the infants tragically died.

This obviously shocked everyone, including Samoan health officials. In the early stages, the cause of death was a mystery – what had caused these two children to die so quickly?

The vaccination program was put on hold while health authorities investigated. If there was an unexpected contaminant, or something unusual about the vaccines, you definitely want to know as soon as possible so the same thing doesn't happen to other children.

They eventually discovered that the MR vaccine itself wasn't the issue, it was the incorrect preparation prior to injection that caused the problem. The two nurses pleaded guilty to manslaughter and were sentenced to at least five years in jail.[4]

However, questions and rumours circulated within the Samoan community regarding the vaccines and even about how the immunisation program was being conducted. In the aftermath, some Samoan parents didn't have the same confidence to vaccinate their kids anymore.[5]

During the time the immunisation program was stalled, childhood vaccination rates dramatically fell, dropping to only twenty-eight per cent by the end of 2018.[6]

The measles vaccination program was eventually reinstated, but with extreme caution. A doctor was required to be present for each vaccination to take place, but this made it difficult to resume the program at the same speed as before the crisis, as there were only a limited number of doctors available.

It was nine months before the program was fully up and running, but families were still dubious.

The stage was set for disaster.

●

Taylor Winterstein is what many Australians would call a WAG – a demeaning acronym for 'Wives and Girlfriends', used predominantly when referring to the partners of famous sportsmen. Her husband, Frank Winterstein, is a prominent NRL footballer, well known in both Australia and Samoa. Taylor's relationship with Frank has propelled her to celebrity status, allowing her to build influence and a significant social media profile.

(As a side note, I'd just like to mention that, for some reason, male partners of sportsmen and sportswomen aren't commonly called HABs, but I'll leave you to come to your own conclusion about why that might be.)

The anti-vaccination movement has been bubbling along for a while around the world and Taylor has joined their ranks. She's frequently spoken out against vaccines and has targeted the Samoan population specifically with misinformation over the years. She has undermined public health campaigns and this contributed to the health crisis seen in Samoa.

In June 2019, Taylor Winterstein travelled to Samoa planning to hold an anti-vaccine workshop titled 'Making Informed Choices' in the capital, Apia. Tickets were A$200 each, but the workshop was cancelled following criticism from the head of the Health Ministry.

However, while there Taylor met with Robert F Kennedy Junior, another well-known anti-vaxxer from the US. She instagrammed a message to her followers, singing the praises of her newfound friend and saying that he was going to change the course of history.[7]

It was not long after this meeting that disaster struck. Samoa recorded its first case of the start of an horrendous measles outbreak in September 2019.[8]

The original case was believed to have come from a New Zealand traveller, and with only low numbers of children vaccinated the Samoan population were left exposed and vulnerable to this potentially deadly viral infection. It spread throughout the community within weeks, and hospitals soon began to overflow at over three hundred per cent capacity. By 15 November 2019 the Samoan Government called a state of emergency.

As Samoa grappled with this epidemic, Taylor posted her disagreement with this announcement on Instagram. Her opinion was that calling a state of emergency and mandatory MMR (measles, mumps and rubella) vaccines for the entire population was the worst possible result.[9]

Samoa was in turmoil, but Taylor continued to post messages downplaying the role of immunisations and spearheaded an anti-vaccination campaign. Her missives only served to muddy the waters and confuse Samoan parents in a crisis.

Her celebrity status enabled her to be influential in discouraging Samoans from immunising their children. As health professionals were scrambling to cope with hospitals well over capacity, her social media posts continued to undermine their work.

Samoan health authorities were determined to stop things from getting worse. In response to the crisis, the government essentially shut down the whole country and embarked on a broad-sweeping vaccination campaign. People were unable to gather outside in groups – not unlike many people's experience during the COVID-19 pandemic that would impact the world only months later.

Taylor Winterstein compared the lockdown to Nazi Germany and ridiculed the government for shipping in vaccinations instead of vitamin A, which is not a proven treatment for measles infection.

In fact, in the middle of the outbreak, the director of the WHO's immunisation department Kate O'Brien noted that the work of anti-vaccination activists had unfortunately been effective and was having 'a very remarkable impact on the immunisation program'.[10]

It seems surreal, but at the time families who weren't vaccinated against measles were asked to hang red flags on the door of their homes so health authorities could come and administer vaccinations to the household members.

It was a mammoth effort and by 29 December 2019, more than ninety-five per cent of the population were immunised allowing Samoa to start returning to normal life again.

But by that point, every village had been impacted. More than 5700 people had been infected and by 22 January 2020 eighty-three people had died.

The Ministry of Health Director-General for Samoa, Leausa Dr Take Naseri, described Taylor Winterstein's campaign as a 'public health threat'. Prime Minister Tuilaepa Dr Sailele Malielegaoi became increasingly frustrated with the unfolding epidemic and spoke out against anti-vaccination campaigners.

Tuilaepa spoke directly to the media about other misinformation too: 'I urge those who are avoiding [getting vaccinated] and going to traditional healers, that those treatments will not cure your measles,' he explained, 'not getting your child immunised is a sign that you are willing to infect your own child.'[11]

While Taylor isn't responsible for what happened, anti-vaccine activists can be dangerous in these situations. They cause confusion in a crisis and have a real-world impact on people's lives. There are many vocal anti-vax types online, all with huge followings – unchecked, they pose a serious threat to society. They can also undermine attempts to reach herd immunity.

The events in Samoa are a clear example of what can happen when vaccination rates are low. A large number of the population were sitting ducks, susceptible to a severe and highly transmissible respiratory viral infection. This was like piling up a mountain of dry timber on a hot day and lighting a match.

As I mentioned before, herd immunity is a term used to describe a situation where enough members of the community have been immunised against an infection, so that it isn't able to spread easily from person to person. It's crucially important because if vaccination rates get too low, the infection is able to sweep through the population causing havoc.

Immunising ninety-five per cent of the community will also protect the five per cent of people who are vulnerable. This includes children who are too young to be immunised yet, patients undergoing chemotherapy, people with weak immune systems, those who are unable to be vaccinated for other medical reasons, and people who may have been vaccinated but the vaccine hasn't sparked a strong enough immune response.

Herd immunity even prevents transmission of infection to anti-vaxxers who choose not to vaccinate themselves and their kids because it protects the people around them. It's ironic that anti-vaxxers benefit from it, while simultaneously trying to undermine it.

Unfortunately, in some places around Australia our vaccination rate is much lower than this target. Low rates of immunity could potentially be okay if people who decided not to immunise their families were spread out evenly around the country but anti-vaxxers tend to cluster together in like-minded groups. This drops the average number of people vaccinated in these local areas and makes them all vulnerable to infection.

In Australia, the main areas of concern for low vaccination rates include the Northern Rivers area along the North Coast of New South Wales, Northern Sydney, Northern Perth, Southern Perth around Fremantle, Central and Eastern Sydney, and some suburban pockets around Melbourne. These areas tend to be more affluent suburbs with young families.

Health messages, like any good public relations exercise, need constant updating in order to get the appropriate information out to the general public. 'Herd immunity' has been used as part of colloquial medical terminology for many decades, but the term has recently been twisted by the anti-vaccination crowd and misinterpreted to take on the opposite meaning of its intention.

Instead of focusing on humanity being all in it together and trying to do the best for ourselves and our neighbours, herd immunity is explained as people 'just going along with the herd' without thinking independently. In other words, we're all mindless 'sheeple' going along with the flock.

In recent years you might have heard health professionals talking about 'community immunity' more than 'herd immunity'; this change in language was designed to reflect that human beings are interlinked and that the decisions we make every day not only affect ourselves and our families but have the potential to affect everyone.

Early in the COVID-19 pandemic, there was a suggestion to let SARS-CoV-2 (the virus that causes you to develop the illness) run rampant through the population in an effort to create herd immunity, but this logic is flawed. Such a strategy would only lead to many people getting sick. This might eventually create herd immunity but you're going to lose a lot of people along the way.

●

Researchers are extremely cautious when they create a vaccine. If you're going to roll out a new immunisation to billions of healthy people around the world, you need to be incredibly confident that it's going to be well tolerated and effective.

By the time I was born in New Zealand the measles vaccination had been around for about a decade. It was introduced as part of the National Immunisation Schedule in 1969, the same year Neil Armstrong set foot on the moon.

While the moon landing may have been a huge moment in history, I would argue the measles vaccination has had much more of an impact on humankind compared to a few steps on the lunar surface.

The rubella (or German measles) vaccination was also introduced to New Zealand around the same time. Rubella usually only causes a mild illness in children and adults but can be devastating for a developing fetus if a pregnant woman is infected.

I thought I was pretty lucky being a boy in New Zealand because one day at primary school all the girls were taken away and lined up to get immunised against rubella. We were told we were exempt from the needle because we couldn't get pregnant.

Later on, it was decided that it was better to immunise both girls and boys to prevent rubella continuing to cycle around the population – so despite not expecting to become pregnant over the course of our lives, the boys eventually got the rubella vaccination anyway.

In 1990, the immunisation for mumps was introduced into the schedule as part of the MMR 'three in one' jab. Mumps is another viral infection that causes the parotid glands in your cheeks to swell up, making it hard to swallow. The infection can also make your testicles or ovaries swollen, potentially causing fertility problems down the track.

My future home across the Tasman Sea had a very similar timeline to the New Zealand program. Measles immunisation was introduced in Australia in 1969, rubella in 1971, mumps in 1981 and eventually the MMR in 1989.

Immunisation rates were high in the early 1990s and prevented millions of deaths from occurring around the world. The number of fetal abnormalities caused by rubella dropped, and as mumps infections decreased, the number of chubby-cheeked children was also on the decline.

This was all great, until Andrew Wakefield entered the scene.

Back in the 1990s, Andrew Wakefield was a practising doctor in the UK who claimed to have discovered that autism spectrum disorder was caused by vaccines. His study got a lot of traction because it was published in the popular medical journal *The Lancet*.

Understandably, this caused parents around the world to panic and many families omitted the MMR vaccination from their program and became more hesitant towards other immunisations too.

In time Wakefield's research was proven to be fraudulent, his conclusion false and the paper was retracted. But the damage had been done. Despite decades of research since and constant reinforcement of messaging around the issue, there are still parents who believe vaccines cause autism. This is just not true.

Part of the problem is that parents of children with autism often notice their child hasn't met their expected developmental milestones at about four years of age – around the same time the MMR vaccination was given. They then came to the false conclusion that the two are connected.

Andrew Wakefield was thoroughly discredited, stripped of his medical registration and shunned by the medical community. He left the UK for the US and was quietly ignored by the media for a number of years.

But in this new age of social media superstardom, his time in the shadows has come to an end. Instead of accepting the criticism of his research, he has doubled down on his original position. His paper continues to be cited in internet echo chambers, despite being retracted from *The Lancet*, and he occasionally pops up in podcasts with people like former celebrity chef Pete Evans.

Pete Evans has provided this discredited man with a platform to further promote his ideas. This gives Wakefield the opportunity to dissuade parents from immunising their children against potentially lethal infections.

Nicole Rogerson is the CEO of Autism Awareness Australia and I asked her about Andrew and Pete.

She said, 'Both of them have played a different but equally reprehensible role in pushing misinformation to parents. Wakefield displayed the most cynical and poor clinical judgement, and he quite rightly has earnt the pariah status he currently enjoys.'

She continued, 'Pete Evans is a different creature. He isn't a clinician and he doesn't have an intellectual or academic background to support his assertions. [He] appeal[s] to a certain (small and often affluent) community of people vulnerable to pseudoscience and nonsense. Normally I would just write these people off intellectually, but sadly Facebook and Instagram have become amplifying platforms which allow them to push the message to new audiences.'

This is the problem – the dangers they pose are serious, and they have a wide reach. I asked Nicole what effect she believes Andrew Wakefield has had on the community and she explained, 'The harm has been significant. I mean this was all twenty years ago and we are still talking about it.' Adding, 'He is promoting ideas that have been directly contradicted by science and evidence and has the thin veil of "conspiracy" cloaked all over it. Sowing the seeds of doubt in the back of parents' minds, which led to the delay and in some cases refusal of parents vaccinating their children.'

I wondered if this controversy had affected vaccination rates in children with autism. Nicole said that a number of parents weren't following the immunisation schedule for their children.

A significant problem she found was that 'parents who had a child with autism may not openly admit to being an anti-vaxxer but they wouldn't vaccinate their younger children "just in case". You have to understand the damage this movement did to parents. I'll admit being nervous as hell the day I took my youngest son into the GP for his shots. Here I was, a sensible educated woman who knew Wakefield had been discredited, but there was still something in the back of my mind. Those mind games are terrible and have reverberated through my community for two decades. Shame on those who continue to push it.'

I asked Nicole how she discusses the science of vaccination with parents of children with ASD who might be worried. She explained, 'To be honest, you need to lead by example and educate rather than lecture. Most parents just desperately want what is best for their child [but] they have been fed a lie and they are vulnerable to the message.

'Lecturing and making people feel dumb won't work. Hear their fears, understand them and help them make the right choice. I am sure I fail a lot and I will admit to having close friends, whose children are now adults, who still believe that vaccinations caused autism. I love them enough to leave the subject alone but I blame Wakefield for their pain.'

Nicole also mentioned, 'One more thing. It is important to understand how offensive Pete Evans is to our community. He is essentially telling parents that autism is so bad, they should risk their child's life at any cost to avoid it. Imagine how that makes our children with autism feel.'

And anti-vaxxers are trying to spread these messages across the country. Andrew Wakefield directed the anti-vaccination propaganda film, *Vaxxed*, which masquerades as a documentary and alleges that there is a major cover-up regarding modern vaccinations and their impact on children. Anti-vaccination communities wishing to broadcast it to Australian audiences have struggled to find cinema locations willing to screen the film because thankfully many theatres across the country have chosen not to be associated with it.

As a result, a large *Vaxxed* bus was driven across the country, spreading a message of misinformation, fear and division.

Nicole has been active in the campaign against the *Vaxxed* film and bus. She said, 'I am a proponent of free speech, but these guys push their luck. It is propaganda, pure and simple. They have a message, a brand and now a roadshow. I may not be able to stop them but I do enjoy tweeting councils and local politicians in the areas they park and set up in. Getting them moved on is a personal professional highlight.'

Another film in this self-described 'documentary' genre is *Sacrificial Virgins*, released in 2017. This film attempts to find a tenuous link (where there is none) between the administration of the HPV vaccine and young women experiencing rare neurological conditions.

The HPV vaccination is very effective at protecting against cervical cancer in women and penile cancer in men. It also decreases the chance of developing head and neck cancers, anal cancer and genital warts. Since the HPV vaccination has been introduced we've seen that it's well tolerated, has few side effects, and hasn't increased the rate of people developing rare neurological disorders.

Eating breakfast is common and getting hit by a car is rare. Just because you ate breakfast and then were hit by a car, doesn't mean that it was your breakfast that caused the car accident. In the same way, HPV vaccination is commonly administered and some neurological conditions are rare. Just because you had an HPV vaccination, doesn't mean it caused the rare neurological condition. Unfortunately, you were probably going to get it anyway.

And it's not just your reproductive tract that's affected by HPV. There are more than one hundred and sixty different types of Human Papilloma Virus; some like to grow on the soles of your feet, others like your fingers and some like to attach themselves closely to your external genitals. Some are raised, some are flat, some you can hardly see and some cause cancer. Nearly one hundred per cent of cervical cancer is caused by these viruses.

In 2007 I was working at a clinic in Melbourne when I first discovered a new HPV vaccination was coming out. It was distributed to medical centres across the country with the clear intention to vaccinate young women, and it was also distributed to schools to immunise young girls.

It was groundbreaking to think that so much suffering from cervical cancer could be avoided by three rounds of this new injection.

The developers were confident there would be minimal side effects as this vaccine had been tested thoroughly. But as it was rolled out there was an issue that kept coming up.

A vasovagal reaction – otherwise known as fainting.

Initially I was concerned – what mechanism of the vaccine could possibly cause someone to collapse after having the needle? Eventually the problem became clear: it wasn't the vaccination, but the population.

Whole classrooms of twelve-year-old girls were lining up to have the needle, one after another. Unfortunately, if one girl fainted or rumours spread about how painful the needle was going to be, then the students' stress levels would collectively rise. They would start feeling anxious in the queue and when it came time for the actual shot, they were much more likely to faint. And if one person fainted, everyone fainted.

But this was easily fixed. By removing the queues and not vaccinating one after another in plain sight, the waiting students' stress levels decreased and so did the rates of fainting.[12]

Following this, cervical cancer rates started to fall and the number of young people affected by genital warts was decreasing, then in 2013 we started immunising boys around Australia too. This was done to prevent boys from transmitting the infection to women, but also to decrease genital warts, penile cancer, anal cancer, and head and neck cancers in men too.

The impact of the HPV vaccine, in combination with a refreshed cervical screening program has been so successful in Australia that we are now expecting cervical cancer to become practically eliminated by 2028.[13]

But while Australia has been extremely successful in preventing HPV infections, Japan and Denmark haven't been going so well, again thanks to the work of anti-vaxxers.

In Japan, a misinformation campaign surrounding the vaccine was successful in halting the rollout in 2013 following the reporting of adverse reactions in the media. These adverse reactions were overblown, with unconfirmed videos of young women having seizures broadcast on the news. As a result, the public was scared, and the vaccination regimen has not been successful. A study published in *The Lancet* in 2020 estimated the hesitancy had resulted in an additional 5000 deaths.[14]

A similar situation in Denmark has required the government to make a concentrated effort to dispel myths and concerns surrounding the HPV vaccine.

Across the world, this work is made so much harder by people with a profile who share misinformation. There are many people with public profiles in Australia – actors, actresses, sports stars, influencers, role models – who have articulated ignorant opinions about vaccinations.

I'd like to think that celebrities don't have much power when it comes to public health, but they can carry a lot of influence, especially if people are undecided or sitting on the fence when it comes to the decision whether to vaccinate.

The best way to handle anti-vaccination activists is tricky, and Julie Leask expressed that her own solution was a bit unconventional, 'that you kind of let sleeping dogs lie'. She said, 'The anti-vax movement is a bit like having a wasp's nest on the side of your house. If you poke a stick at it, you'll make it worse, but if you recognise it's just there, buzzing away then you can just ignore it.'

Julie stated that her 'strategy of dealing with the anti-vaccination activists is not to feed the trolls, to give them as little attention as possible. Unless they're possibly going to have an impact. Like for example where they might try to stand outside a school gate handing out flyers.'

The group formerly known as the Australian Vaccination Network (AVN) was started up many years ago in the Northern Rivers area, on the North Coast of New South Wales, as a lobby group.

The AVN had the potential to cause harm. They were inappropriately named and questioning parents could be lured to their website when googling information about vaccines. The work of grass roots campaigners and sceptical organisations in Australia, like Stop the Australian Vaccination Network, were effective in having the group change their name, and prevented the anti-vaccination group from being as effective as they could have been.

Those who do guerilla work to combat this misinformation deserve credit.

In that Northern Rivers region, a group of concerned locals got together to battle the anti-vaccine beliefs that surrounded them. In a region with the lowest vaccination rates in the country, the Northern Rivers Vaccination Supporters was designed as a safe space online for parents and others living in the area to get science-based information or have a friendly non-judgemental chat with others who are well versed in the latest science.

Their work has been recognised and their website was endorsed by the WHO as a reputable source of information on the topic.

And then of course there is the information from official sources, like the Department of Health and Ageing, who have published a booklet you can read online for free, called *Myths and Realities – Responding to Arguments Against Vaccination.*[15]

It's a wealth of information on immunisations, but it's unlikely to convince anyone belonging to an anti-vaccination cult – they aren't big fans of trusting government departments.

The evidence in support of vaccinations is overwhelming and our knowledge and expertise continues to grow. In August 2020, it was announced that Africa is now free of wild polio for the first time, as more than ninety-five per cent of the population has been immunised. This is an incredible milestone that has saved lives, pain and difficulties for countless numbers of people.

The scientific community has taken dramatic steps with vaccination technology, including the ability to roll out new influenza vaccinations each year to match the strains likely to cause the most trouble. The COVID-19 pandemic stepped everything up a notch with messenger RNA (mRNA) and double-stranded DNA (dsDNA) vaccines now able to provide a quick turnaround for updating immunisations and enabling us to parallel changes in viral mutations.

Infections kill people, vaccines save lives.

CHAPTER 14

COOKED

Australians love reality television and in the 2010s we had a particular penchant for cooking shows. Set up a cooktop, turn on the timer and dial up the heat with a bit of friendly competition – we just couldn't get enough.

MasterChef was a ratings success for Network Ten in 2009, but Channel 7 wasn't far behind in 2010 with *My Kitchen Rules* co-hosted by celebrity chefs, Pete Evans and Manu Feildel.

The concept for *My Kitchen Rules* was relatively simple. Teams from around Australia (and New Zealand) competed to make their homes into restaurants while fellow contestants judged their efforts.

Seasons spanning from 2010 to 2020 dominated our television screens. The grand final episodes scored a rating in the top ten most watched television events from 2012 to 2016 and in 2013 achieved top position as the most watched event on Australian television. *MKR*, as it was affectionately known, even won a Logie Award in 2014 for the most popular reality television show.[1]

At the start of the decade, the co-hosts were suddenly shot into the limelight and their popularity skyrocketed as the seasons continued.

Manu Feildel was bestowed with an elegant French accent that could melt anyone's croque madame, and Pete Evans was charming, charismatic with roguish good looks and appeared genuinely keen to educate others about healthy eating.

In November 2012, Pete Evans contributed to *Sunday Life* magazine (which ran in the major papers *The Sunday Age* and *The Sun-Herald*) with 'My Day on a Plate'. This was meant to be a list of the typical foods he would consume each day from dawn to dusk, and his culinary style immediately became an internet meme overnight.[2]

Pete's day started with a couple of glasses of alkalised water, organic spirulina, maca, activated almonds and coconut kefir, with dinner including cultured vegetables, emu meatballs and liquorice root tea.

This was an unusual grocery list for most Australians. It raised a few eyebrows and 'activated almonds' suddenly became a popular phrase around the country. Raw almonds are 'activated' by placing them in water for a few hours. This encourages them to germinate (get ready to sprout) and is said to make them more easily digested.

Pete Evans was widely criticised on social media for his dietary habits, and you could probably say this was an overreaction as Pete wasn't hurting anyone by choosing to eat damp food.

'My Day on a Plate' was one of the first public glimpses of Pete Evans' quirky behaviour, but this was just a taste of things to come.

FLUORIDE

In December 2014, Pete travelled to Western Australia to meet up with an anti-fluoride lobby group called Fluoride Free, who were campaigning to remove the mineral from drinking water.

Scientific evidence shows that water is safe to drink and is effective at decreasing tooth decay when it contains small amounts of fluoride. However, Pete Evans described fluoride as a 'neurotoxin' and stated that he never touched tap water. He was concerned that fluoride could be a major contributor towards 'thyroid, brain and degenerative diseases'.[3]

Australian Medical Association (AMA) Western Australian President, Dr Michael Gannon, responded to Pete's concerns by saying, 'It's always disappointing when people use their celebrity in a way that is not useful to society. In cases like this, when people are simply wrong, we ask that they butt out of the debate.'

Dr Gannon continued, 'Water fluoridation is something that has the full backing of the Australian Dental Association and the AMA. It's cheap, it's proven to be beneficial and data repeatedly proves that it is effective in reducing cavities in children.'[4]

Dr Matthew Hopcraft is a dentist, academic researcher, and an Associate Professor at Melbourne Dental School. He's also in favour of fluoride being in our drinking water. He is very familiar with the opinions of anti-fluoride activists like Pete Evans and Fluoride Free, but he doesn't find their arguments convincing.

Dr Hopcraft has been involved with research on the impact of water fluoridation on tooth decay in Australian adults, has published his research in peer-reviewed scientific journals, and has been involved in developing Australia's guidelines on water fluoridation.[5]

I contacted Matt and asked for his insights on the issue. He explained, 'There have been a large number of studies that show water fluoridation to be safe and effective around the world. Studies that show [detrimental] health effects are either animal studies, often with higher concentrations of fluoride, or are based in parts of the world where high levels of fluoride naturally occur [in the water] – upwards of 4–10 ppm [parts per million].'

Drinking a concentrated amount of fluoride has the potential to cause harm, but Matt reassuringly told me, 'We adjust the amount of fluoride in tap water to around 1 ppm in Australia.' This very low concentration is proven to be safe.

Water fluoridation began in Tasmania in 1953 with the major cities coming on board later – Sydney and Perth in 1968, Adelaide in 1971, Darwin in 1972 and Melbourne in 1977. Brisbane remained unfluoridated until 2008.

'There is no evidence of adverse health outcomes in the rest of the country compared to Brisbane over 40 years,' Matt told me. 'This is one of the strongest arguments to demonstrate safety – if there were adverse health outcomes, we would have expected to see this comparing Brisbane to Sydney, Melbourne, Perth and Adelaide over that period.'

In 2017, the National Health and Medical Research Council (NHMRC) reviewed the depth and breadth of scientific evidence and provided a statement about fluoridation of our water supply. They concluded that 'water fluoridation reduces tooth decay by 26–44% in children and adolescents, and by 27% in adults'.[6]

The NHMRC looked for evidence of possible adverse health effects from fluoridated water and concluded:

> There is reliable evidence that community water fluoridation at current Australian levels is not associated with cancer, Down syndrome, cognitive dysfunction, lowered intelligence or hip fracture. There is no reliable evidence of an association between community water fluoridation at current Australian levels and other human health conditions such as chronic kidney disease, kidney stones, hardening of the arteries (atherosclerosis), high blood pressure, low birth weight, all-cause mortality, musculoskeletal pain, osteoporosis, skeletal fluorosis, thyroid problems or self-reported ailments such as gastric discomfort, headache and insomnia.[7]

It's pretty clear that the NHMRC addressed all of the issues raised by Pete Evans and Fluoride Free, but instead of listening to these public health experts, Pete has doubled down on his anti-fluoride stance. He has offered little supportive evidence to explain his point of view and simply recommends for his supporters to do their own research.

Despite holding these unusual ideas about public health, his regular appearances on television allowed his popularity to grow. His range of cookbooks were a huge success and in part thanks to him the Paleo diet was touted as an excellent way of getting fit, healthy and losing weight.

PALEO FOR KIDS

In 2015 Pete Evans co-authored a cookbook titled *Bubba Yum Yum: The Paleo Way for New Mums, Babies and Toddlers*, but it never made it to the shelves.

The reason was shocking. The Dietitians Association of Australia (DAA) assessed the cookbook prior to its release and published a media alert stating that some of the recipes contained within the cookbook were potentially lethal, especially for children.

The DAA were particularly concerned about a DIY infant formula made from liver, cod liver oil and bone broth found in the book. Their media alert stated that the 'DIY [infant] formula is said to be comparable to breast milk, but the analysis proves this is not the case'. Their findings showed, 'It is significantly higher than breast milk in Vitamin A (749% higher), Vitamin B12 (2326% higher), protein (220% higher), iron (1067% higher), sodium (879% higher) and a range of other nutrients.'

The DAA concluded, 'This formula could be very harmful to infants [and] their immature immune and digestive systems could not cope with this formulation'. They were concerned for newborn babies because 'the formulation could cause permanent damage and possibly result in death'.[8]

Newborn babies have complex dietary needs and the Australian infant feeding guidelines promote breastfeeding as a priority. If breastmilk is not available (for whatever reason) using a commercially produced infant formula is the only suitable and safe alternative.[9]

Baby formula is a great scientific achievement. Infants can die if they don't receive the correct combination of nutrients, but thanks to science, baby formula contains exactly the right ingredients to keep them alive when breastmilk isn't available.

Publishing a cookbook that encourages people to create their own baby formula from bone broth and liver is a bold move and the Department of Health was alerted to the potential dangers of this publication. They reviewed the recipes and were also concerned about the nutritional content.[10]

The President of the Public Health Association of Australia, Heather Yeatman, said at the time, 'In my view, there's a very real possibility that a baby may die if this book goes ahead.'[11]

Dr Nikki Stamp, a cardiothoracic surgeon with an interest in 'health' advice posted online, described the *Bubba Yum Yum* recipe book as 'downright dangerous, arrogant and bordering on criminal'.[12]

In response, the publisher, Pan Macmillan, decided not to release the book, but Pete and his co-authors, blogger Charlotte Carr and naturopath Helen Padarin, were determined to publish it digitally.

They tweaked their baby bone broth recipe and renamed it, but when they returned to present their brand new broth, it still contained vitamin A at toxic levels. At least they had decreased the amount from ten, to now only four and a half times the maximum acceptable daily limit.[13] This is better but still not ideal.

The DAA responded again with a further media alert cautioning parents about the DIY infant formula now called 'Happy Tummy Brew'. The DAA stated:

> The authors seem to have made a serious mistake with this second version of their liver and broth recipe, suggesting they do not understand the basic scientific and nutrition information relevant for infant feeding. They have said publicly that they have tried to make it safe by reworking the original recipe, and increasing the age for which it's suggested from 0-6 months to 6-12 months, but they have failed spectacularly to meet any safe standards. This new infant 'brew' could seriously harm babies.[14]

Unfortunately, we had just climbed the foothills and hadn't yet reached the mountain of misinformation Pete was preparing to deliver to his audience.

SUNSCREEN AND SUN-GAZING

My first interaction with Pete Evans came early one morning in July 2016. My phone rang while I was eating breakfast, and I answered to a friendly producer from a local Sydney breakfast radio show *Fitzy & Wippa*.

The producer explained that Fitzy and Wippa were keen to have me on air to discuss Pete Evans' latest controversy – his comments about sunscreen.

Just days earlier, one of the chef's Facebook followers, a group which he calls his tribe, had asked what he used for sunscreen. He revealed that he didn't usually wear any sunscreen at all and suggested it was silly for people to 'put on normal chemical sunscreen then lay out in the sun for hours on end and think they are safe because they have covered themselves in poisonous chemicals'.[15]

The response from the Cancer Council had been swift. They reminded everyone that regular use of sunscreen is safe and has been proven to significantly reduce the risk of developing skin cancer.[16]

Pete was right to say that relying on sunscreen alone won't guarantee your protection from sunburn or skin cancer. It's important to use a variety of methods to avoid harmful sunlight exposure, but discouraging people from using sunscreen as part of our armament goes against all of our important and successful public health campaigns.

The producer told me they would speak with Pete Evans first and then get me on the line afterwards to provide clarity on the science, but what happened next was a bit of a kerfuffle.

Instead of having us on the show at different times, I was dropped into the middle of Fitzy and Wippa's conversation with Pete and they expected us to fight it out over the airwaves.

After listening to Pete's concerns, I calmly stated the scientific facts and encouraged listeners to continue wearing sunscreen. Pete raised his voice to discourage sunscreen use and I raised mine in rebuttal.

My partner, unaware of what was happening, came rushing down the stairs to find out why I was shouting about the rates of skin cancer in Australia so early in the morning.

GPs like myself spend a significant amount of time treating sun-damaged skin with cryotherapy (liquid nitrogen), preventing these areas from turning into skin cancers. We're also trained to perform skin biopsies and excise skin lesions, a medical skill that saves our patients' lives.

Australia has one of the highest rates of skin cancer in the world. According to the Cancer Council, we're two to three times more likely to develop it over our lives compared with people living in Canada, the US and the UK. It's a frightening statistic that two out of three Australians will develop skin cancer by the time they are seventy years old.[17]

It's for this reason that hearing Pete plant seeds of doubt about sunscreen into the minds of radio listeners was so frustrating. Our well-known public health campaign has taken decades to build, but even casual remarks from a popular figure can undermine this good work. Pete may not appreciate the gravity of this situation because he hasn't had to cut chunks of cancer out of people's skin.

Sunscreen is a turn-off if it's sticky, greasy or smelly, but our 'Slip! Slop! Slap!' campaign has been highly successful in making the public aware of the dangers of prolonged sunlight exposure and teaching everyone how to protect themselves.

Since the campaign began in 1981 and Sid the Seagull became a household name, rates of melanoma in younger Australians have fallen steadily, while those in older Australians have risen slightly – as they continue to pay for the sun-loving culture of their younger years.[18]

In 2016, after thirty-five years of SunSmart messaging, you can understand why organisations like the Cancer Council get a bit touchy when Pete Evans tells the public that sunscreen is poisonous.

Sunscreen is made of chemicals that either reflect and scatter ultraviolet light (such as zinc oxide and titanium dioxide) or absorb and neutralise it before it reaches your skin (such as oxybenzone and octinoxate).

The suggestion that sunscreen contains poisonous chemicals plays on the fear that sunscreen could be harmful if your body soaked it up like a sponge, but most of the chemicals don't get absorbed. They remain on your skin until they gradually wash off. Small amounts may penetrate through the skin and enter your body, but these haven't been found to cause harm. What's much more likely to cause harm if it gets into your body is metastatic skin cancer.

However, the Cancer Council's SunSmart program has never just been about sunscreen. 'Slip on a shirt, slop on sunscreen and slap on a hat' became a well-known phrase across the country and was a reminder that we needed a multi-pronged approach against harmful ultraviolet light. In 2007, the slogan was updated to 'Slip, slop, slap, seek, slide' to encourage seeking shade and sliding on some sunglasses.

In December 2018, when I happened to be lathered in sunscreen at the beach, I saw Pete had written an Instagram message to his tribe extolling the virtues of swimming in ocean water and taking a 'brief gaze into the radiant light of the early rising or late setting Sun'.[19]

Pete may be right about one thing – open water swimming can work wonders for some people's mental and physical health, but the same can't be said for gazing directly at the sun.

Sun-gazing was made popular in the 1960s by Hira Ratan Manek in India. The theory is that if you stand on the ground with bare feet and stare at the sun, your body will be recharged by the sun's energy.

Somehow.

You might be surprised to learn that science is yet to prove this.

My parents were militant about the need to wear sunglasses. In their minds, living under the harsh, unforgiving Australian sun was sure to blind us all, especially after coming from our lives in Wellington, where dark storm clouds provided sunlight protection for most of the year.

Your vision is precious and looking directly into the sun should be avoided no matter where in the world you are. If you're not careful your cornea and lens will converge and concentrate the sun's rays onto the retina at the back of your eye. This isn't a good thing.

When I was a kid, the clouds in Wellington would occasionally part and we'd have a nice day. That's when I'd usually entertain myself by going into the backyard with a magnifying glass and burning my name into the timber fence. I'd focus the sunlight into a tiny beam that wasn't strong enough to set the fence on fire (which my neighbours were happy about) but was powerful enough to singe a few letters into the dry wood.

The lens and cornea at the front of your eyes also work like this magnifying glass. If I can burn my name into a wooden fence, just imagine what the same focused rays of sunlight could do to your retina.

Ophthalmologists frequently care for patients who have watched eclipses without wearing eye protection. Examining the patients' retina reveals burnt areas in the shape of fingernail clippings where the sun has permanently etched its signature. This phenomenon is called solar retinopathy and can cause permanent loss of vision in the affected area.[20]

All injuries to the eye are taken seriously because once your vision is gone, it can be gone forever. Even a brief gaze at the sun can cause lasting effects on your eyesight.

Prolonged sunlight exposure over your lifetime also speeds up the development of cataracts, when the normally clear lens in the eye becomes clouded. More than seventy per cent of Australians over eighty years old will develop the condition. Fortunately we have access to successful treatment, and cataract surgery is one of the most commonly performed operations in this country, where the clouded lens is replaced with a brand new artificial one.[21]

DAIRY-FREE

Elderly Australians are also more likely to have low bone density. The Australian Institute of Health and Welfare estimates that osteoporosis affects twenty-nine per cent of women and ten per cent of men over seventy-five years of age, putting them at an increased risk of bone fractures.[22]

Osteoporosis is potentially catastrophic – just the slightest trip, bump or fall can result in a fracture. In August 2016, one of Pete's tribe asked for some dietary advice, saying they had been diagnosed with osteoporosis and wanted to know if the Paleo diet would help.

Pete advised him to remove dairy products from his diet because 'calcium from dairy can remove calcium from your bones', adding 'most doctors do not know this information'.[23]

He got one thing right – most doctors do not know this information. My medical colleagues didn't know it, I didn't know it and when I asked Professor Peter Ebeling, endocrinologist and medical director of Osteoporosis Australia, even he didn't know it – because it's blatantly preposterous.

Peter told me, 'I think most doctors would realise his claim about calcium from dairy removing calcium from bones was misinformation,' but unfortunately 'the lay public would not [know it was untrue] and would believe him due to his celebrity status.'

The peak health authorities for osteoporosis in Australasia are the Australian and New Zealand Bone and Mineral Society, Osteoporosis Australia and the Endocrine Society of Australia. At the time of Pete's claims about dairy, these leading organisations responded by publishing a joint statement on the benefits of dietary calcium, clearly rejecting Pete's suggestion that the calcium contained within dairy foods could draw out calcium from your bones.

'Pete Evans' actions highlight the danger of celebrities without medical training commenting on public health issues,' Peter opined. 'I wonder how many fractures and deaths resulted from self-interested actions?'

Bad health advice, even when dished out with good intentions, has the power to cause harm. Pete Evans isn't a doctor and it's understandable that he might make the odd mistake when he's speaking online or in the media. However, once you've been corrected by multiple leading health authorities and informed of the facts, it's unacceptable to continue repeating the same misinformation to your fans.

It's disheartening to see this process in action, where popular figures lack the cognitive capacity to stop themselves spreading misinformation on social media. Instead of showing humility and learning from their mistakes, celebrities often dig their heels in, determined to be right despite the facts.

All this dangerous health advice was being peddled by Pete Evans, while he was one of the biggest television stars in the country.

STIRRING THE POT

Channel 7 continued to put him on television screens each week, despite his outrageous health claims off camera. Keeping him as a judge on their most successful prime-time show provided him with a thin veneer of credibility and gave him a national platform. While not explicitly endorsing him, they were giving him a voice and essentially saying his opinion was worthy of our time and attention.

Pete Evans kept pushing the boundaries of reality and in March 2019 he revealed more about his association with the unusual world of anti-vaxxers. On his Facebook page he posted his thanks to a known anti-vaccination campaigner, Sherri Tenpenny, for asking 'the questions that need to be asked about vaccines and medicine'.[24]

The President of the Australian Medical Association at the time, Dr Tony Bartone, responded by saying, 'When it comes to cooking, Pete Evans might be an expert, but his misinformation about vaccination is a recipe for disaster.'[25]

When the controversies became too big to ignore Channel 7 washed their hands of Paleo Pete and parted ways with him in 2020.

But the damage was done. Pete had already built an extensive social media following of loyal fans and continued to leverage his popularity for influence and money.

In addition to his line of cookbooks, he diversified with a range of products including vitamins, probiotic drinks, a range of vinegars, sauces, fermented mustards, pet foods, water filters, moisturisers, magnets, infrared lights and mats, restaurants, essential oils and in 2020 he started selling a fancy light called a Biocharger.

The lamp's price tag was an incredible US$15,000, which Pete claimed could be used for the 'Wuhan Coronavirus' in a Facebook live stream.[26]

The Therapeutic Goods Administration stated that Pete Evans' health claim had 'no apparent foundation'. His company was issued with two infringement notices, totalling A$25,200, for making alleged advertising breaches both in the Facebook live stream and also on his website.[27]

This didn't prevent him from opening a healing clinic in 2020, located in Byron Bay, that features a hot chamber, a cold chamber and a hyperbaric chamber.

He's even engaged with the development of an 'off-matrix' community situated on a 3500-acre (1400-hectare) block of land in the Northern Rivers area of New South Wales. This area of the world has seen its fair share of spiritual leaders and harmful cults in the past, so hopefully Pete Evans' segregated commune doesn't fall into this category in the future.

Previously when he was under contract with Channel 7, he appeared to temper some of his views, but after this contract ended his opinions have become more extreme. He no longer camouflages his concern about vaccines by saying he's 'just asking questions'. Now he regularly interviews well-known anti-vaccination campaigners and conspiracy theorists on his podcast. One of his guests has been David Icke, who you may already know as the ex-footballer who theorised the world was run by a race of shapeshifting reptilian aliens who live in human form and have infiltrated our governments. Although some of our leaders may appear to be reptilian in nature, David Icke's theory has never been validated.

Pete Evans has also shared many social media posts relating to QAnon, the disproven conspiracy theory – or what Buzzfeed calls a 'collective delusion' – that the world is run by a cabal of Satan-worshipping paedophiles who have kidnapped hundreds of thousands of children and are keeping them hidden in underground tunnels around the world as part of a global sex-trafficking ring.

Pete Evans shared a post in 2020 claiming the mainstream media would soon be announcing that high-profile individuals had been diagnosed with COVID-19 and this would allegedly be a secret code to mean they had confessed to crimes against humanity and were being prepared for execution – these theories have not come to fruition.[28]

Don't forget, this is a man who just months earlier was the star of a very popular reality show on mainstream Australian television, with a very significant social media following.

For years it felt like the more my colleagues and I complained about the dangers Pete posed to the public, the more he was seen as an entertaining, controversial character who was great for television. But in November 2020 he took a step too far.

He posted on his social media platforms a drawing of a caterpillar speaking with a butterfly. The caterpillar was wearing a MAGA cap, and said to the butterfly, 'You've changed.' The butterfly responded, 'We're supposed to.'

This may appear like an innocent conversational exchange between two creatures but the butterfly wings displayed the Nazi symbol known as Schwarze Sonne, the Black Sun.

A follower commented, 'The symbol on the butterfly is a representation of the black sun lol,' to which Pete replied, 'I was waiting for someone to see that.'[29]

The backlash was understandable. Multiple companies who carried Pete's products began distancing themselves from him. Pan Macmillan stated they were going to go their separate ways. Dymocks Booksellers declared they would no longer stock his books and offered a refund to anyone who wanted to return their purchases. Baccarat, Coles and many other brands also announced that they were going to disengage from their association with him and his company.[30]

These business decisions weren't made lightly, but they should have happened much earlier. A man who poses a danger to public health should not be gracing our television screens every night, should not be endorsing products in our supermarkets nor should he be publishing books to be displayed on bookshop shelves.

Pete Evans had a track record of providing bad health advice that could cause real harm, so why was he still presenting a prime-time television show? He campaigned against fluoride, sunscreen, cow's milk, WiFi, 5G and vaccinations. He encouraged sun-gazing and tried to sell expensive fluorescent lamps to handle the 'Wuhan Coronavirus' that he also said was a hoax.

Yet he was still given a platform. It wasn't until a cartoon depicting a Nazi symbol was posted on his social media that his sponsors finally decided to pull the plug.

This isn't about denying someone their freedom of speech or cancelling them because we don't like their ideas. This is about deplatforming a person with influence in order to prevent them from causing more harm.

Social media corporations must also shoulder some of the responsibility here. They have the ability to prevent misinformation and disinformation from spreading on their platforms, but previously didn't have the impetus to do so. It wasn't until the end of 2020 that Facebook finally decided to remove Pete's page from the site for sharing misinformation about coronavirus.

Too little too late.

When major media organisations provide celebrities with airtime, they also lend them credibility. We tend to trust the people chosen to grace our screens, but confidence doesn't make you right.

Charismatic conspiracy theorists might attract attention, ratings and money for the network, but then it's our society who pays the price.

It would be simple if our media organisations were trusted to present us with truthful advice, but the deluge of scientific-sounding healthiness on our television, radio and social media feeds makes it difficult to sift fact from fiction. Unfortunately, at this point of human history, it's still up to you to determine what's true and who to trust.

Be inquisitive and curious about your health. Ask questions and be prepared to change your view depending on scientific evidence.

Seek health advice from a qualified health professional and think twice before investing your time and money in a quick-fix cure.

Critical thinking is vital. It's the only way to stop being a sucker for bad advice and prevent yourself from getting hoodwinked by charlatans with pretty eyes and a great Instagram filter.

Learning basic principles of science and medicine takes time, but it's not hard to take a step back and think, 'Why am I taking sunscreen advice from a chef ... and why on earth am I staring at the sun?'

CHAPTER 15

THE COVID-19 CONSPIRACY

When stories of a novel coronavirus hit the headlines in early 2020, those in the medical profession were optimistic. We'd witnessed similar events in 2002 with SARS (Severe Acute Respiratory Syndrome) and in 2012 with MERS (Middle East Respiratory Syndrome), but these viruses were contained and hadn't spread to pandemic proportions. It was expected this newly identified coronavirus would similarly fade into the background of history.

Therefore, the beginning of the year was like any other – hopeful, happy and full of fireworks.

Then came the COVID-19 pandemic.

With hindsight, this was going to happen eventually. Infectious diseases have plagued humankind forever and it was only a matter of time before a new infection would evolve into a perfect match for causing chaos in our bodies.

But this international event occurred at a time when we're more connected than ever. We watched the virus move from country to country in almost real time, but one thing that spread faster than Severe Acute Respiratory Syndrome Coronavirus 2 (SARS-CoV-2) was the spread of misinformation.

In fact, the amount of false information that needed to be countered was so bad the WHO said they were also battling an 'infodemic' alongside the pandemic.

A new virus that the world has never seen before brings with it a lot of questions – questions that often can't be answered easily or quickly. Fear gripped the world and people started to panic.

In a knowledge vacuum, myths flourish.

As a result, there were misunderstandings, there was gossip, there were deliberate attempts to spread the wrong information, and there were people trying to seize an opportunity to promote their own agendas.

STAGES OF GRIEVING

Whenever you face disappointment, tragedy or life doesn't go in the direction you're quite expecting it to, it's human nature to enter into a state of grief. We all go through our own experience of grieving. There's no right or wrong way to process these emotions either.

The typical stages of grieving include denial, bargaining, anger, depression and eventually acceptance. Suddenly the entire human population was thrown into turmoil. No one was prepared for such an event, and we all had no choice but to change our plans and head into a new, unexpected way of life. As we cancelled weddings, trips overseas and music festivals, we began to grieve the lives we had planned.

And these very normal human emotions are a great way to categorise the odd thoughts some of us had as we tried to process the incredible changes that were occurring around us. For most of us these ideas were fleeting, but for some of us, these thoughts stuck and grew into conspiracy theories as our brains grappled with our new 'COVID-normal'.

Denial

In the very early stages of the pandemic, even the institutions set out to protect us were going through a process of denial. The WHO told people not to panic as they believed there was 'no clear evidence' COVID-19 could be transmitted between humans.[1]

This may not have been complete denial, but it was at least leaning towards an optimistic take on an important issue. We soon discovered this was incorrect. Human-to-human transmission was happening and the WHO quickly took back their statement and started taking the outbreak very seriously.

Unfortunately, this set the stage for uncertainty. People were unsure what to believe, leading to distrust. Just days after being told the virus would be contained within Wuhan, China, we saw it sweep across Italy.

It's not necessarily the WHO's fault – science is messy and during an outbreak what may seem right today is not guaranteed to be true tomorrow. However, conflicting messages only serve to cause confusion.

Around the same time, political leaders were similarly not keen to accept this as their new reality. As the outbreak began in Australia, Prime Minister Scott Morrison told people it was fine to go to the footy that weekend, but that gatherings of over 500 people would be limited from the following week.[2]

We've now seen the consequences of the pandemic play out around the globe – but it can still be difficult to explain an invisible threat to the public.

COVID-19 can only be seen with an electron microscope or detected through technical scientific analysis.[3] For anyone not trained in biological sciences, it can be a stretch to understand the reality of an unseen enemy. A fair bit of trust needs to be placed in the public health authorities telling you that it's a real threat you need to be worried about, and this trust isn't bolstered by inconsistent messages.

Part of denial is just to ignore what's happening – and there were plenty of people who dismissed the threat as nothing more than a hoax. For some it seemed too unreal, like the plot of a terrifying movie.

Social isolation can exacerbate this feeling. If you're bouncing around in your home, staring at the same four walls day after day, I can see how easy it would be to start wondering whether you're being taken for a ride. When people are unable to work and suffering from financial stress with no end in sight, it might seem like it's a big joke and that you're bearing the brunt of it.

Add modern technology into the equation and suddenly groups of like-minded people are finding each other, confirming one another's misconceptions and solidifying their thought processes. Forums flourished with people questioning the official narrative.

If you don't believe you're in danger, you're not going to take precautions.

When health authorities around the world recommended we not gather in large groups, keep a physical distance of 1.5 metres away from each other, wash our hands regularly, use alcohol-based antiseptic gels and wear facial coverings there was some pushback.

Even some people who were in hospital, sick with COVID-19, refused to believe they had the infection. They didn't call their relatives one last time because they thought they would get better. They thought they couldn't die from an infection that didn't exist.[4]

But viruses don't care if you believe in them or not.

Bargaining

Another stage of grief we commonly experience is bargaining.

People everywhere played down the virus, claiming it wasn't really that bad.

Coronaviruses aren't a new phenomenon. They are a family of viruses that typically cause the common cold, so many believed that if they were infected, it was going to affect them in the same way. The virus was also compared with influenza, which can also be pretty nasty – killing 0.1% of the people it infects each year. All up, COVID-19 was estimated to kill approximately one per cent of the people it infected.

This death rate is ten times worse than influenza. Patients with the flu might be placed on a ventilator for a few days until they start recovering, but it's unusual to see them ventilated for more than three weeks, something which is more commonly seen with COVID-19.

The numbers aren't really comparable to COVID-19 though. It was initially estimated that about eighty per cent of people infected with SARS-CoV-2 wouldn't need to go to hospital – this includes people with no symptoms, mild symptoms and moderate symptoms. About twenty per cent were likely to need admission to hospital, with fifteen per cent staying on a general ward and five per cent needing to be ventilated in intensive care.

Proclaiming, wishing or hoping that this novel coronavirus is just like the flu is like saying that a hungry tiger is just like a contented Persian house cat.

People also wanted to bargain with the impact they were willing to let it have on their lives. It was hard to explain to people in the early months of 2020 that it was the start of a marathon, not a sprint. That the infection was bad. And even if you didn't think you'd be terribly affected by it, you just couldn't be sure.

Some people thought that to mitigate the virus we didn't need to lock down whole populations, instead only making our elderly family members hibernate at home while the rest of us walk freely around the streets. With the young having a lower likelihood of dying, shouldn't that be okay?

In countries where such a strategy has taken place and SARS-CoV-2 has been able to run rampant through the community, they've realised just how difficult it is to prevent the virus from getting into elderly populations. When infection rates are soaring and the virus is being transmitted freely by young people who may not even know they are COVID-19 positive, the possibility of it entering a nursing home is extremely high – like a tsunami of virus knocking at the front door just waiting for the right person to let it in. It's just too difficult to protect the elderly sufficiently. The general public simply aren't trained in wearing personal protective equipment and aren't vigilant enough at wearing it. Even if you're taking extreme precautions when you're visiting your nana in a retirement village, you could still transmit the infection to her or to someone else in the facility. And once it's introduced into an unvaccinated elderly population, it spreads like wildfire.

While the majority of people who have died from COVID-19 have been over sixty-five years old, plenty of young people have still ended up on ventilators, have had strokes or have died from the infection.

When we look across the whole population, we just can't tell whether you are the type of person who is going to be fine or one of those people who will become really sick and/or die. It's best not to take your chances with the infection and avoid it until you're able to be vaccinated.

Anger

The next stage of grieving is anger. When our lives are interrupted, it's common to look for someone to blame or find a place to direct our frustration.

The rhetoric from former US President Donald Trump, who called it the 'China virus', is an example of this. Leaders around the world pointed fingers. Some of my own friends and family were even convinced the virus was created in a Chinese laboratory and then slipped out or released on the public. They'd learnt this from watching YouTube videos.

Such a claim has never been proven and a manmade coronavirus is extremely unlikely.

Others wanted to blame technology, and the new 5G communication towers being installed on our street corners became a target. Wuhan was said to be one of the first locations where 5G technology was installed and this was used to explain the origin of the outbreak.[5]

Rumours spread across the internet suggesting signals from 5G towers impaired the immune system, allowing the virus to take hold. There were even claims that coronavirus was purposefully released into the population so 5G could be placed around the city while everyone was in lockdown – which does sound like an elaborate plan. Around the globe, people's anger was directed skyward and in the UK about eighty telecommunication towers were burnt to the ground.[6]

Ironically people working from home or isolated from loved ones needed to be connected more than ever and destroying the towers only served to slow down the internet speed and limit that communication further.

Depression

Another stage of grief is depression, which includes a feeling of everything seeming too hard and wanting to give up.

Some countries found the virus was everywhere very quickly and didn't know what to do about a seemingly insurmountable problem.

In order to keep COVID-19 under control, in small numbers and prevent your hospitals from overflowing, you need to have strong leadership and incredible vigilance, but it seemed that some political leaders let their citizens down by putting their heads in the sand and wishing it would all blow over. But it didn't.

Half-hearted efforts delayed action and a disjointed approach to fighting the pandemic has cost hundreds of thousands of lives around the world. There's no time to feel depressed and take a doona day when you're in the middle of a pandemic.

Acceptance

The final stage of grieving is acceptance. This is when you understand your life is going in a different direction from what you expected, and you begin to comprehend the impact and make plans accordingly. Yet, even among those who accepted the danger, there was still a lot of misinformation in the early days. Panic, desperation and confusion make people vulnerable and gullible enough to make rash decisions – which isn't helped by a rapidly evolving situation.

The WHO was confronted with so much false information being spread online that they found it necessary to make official statements not only about 5G towers, but also the impact of alcohol, antibiotics, bleach, cold weather, hot weather, hand dryers, humidity, hot baths, hot peppers, houseflies, face masks, medication, mosquitoes, salty water, shoes, sunlight, supplements, swimming, thermal scanners, ultra-violet light and vitamins.[7]

That's a lot of confused messages bouncing around the world in a short amount of time.

The number of people promising cures went through the roof. As always, the usual suspects come out – people were consuming more garlic, ginger, vitamin C, vitamin D, zinc supplements or taking probiotics to improve their gut flora. There's a little bit of evidence to suggest that taking zinc supplements for a short period of time may lessen the symptoms when you get a common cold, but it was far too early to know if it did anything to help combat COVID-19.

Even athletic clothing company Lorna Jane was fined almost $40,000 by the TGA for advertising 'anti-virus activewear'.[8]

Adding to the confusion was the early advice from the WHO that they weren't sure face masks would help. This advice changed with new evidence showing masks did limit the spread of infection and public health messages were altered according to these findings. However, some people were already wedded to the original advice and didn't change their tune. It's great to see that people were listening to the WHO to begin with, but it's also important for the general public to keep up to date with a dynamically changing situation.

Following the science is crucial but you need to change your behaviour as new research comes to light.

DIAGNOSIS

The most common symptoms for COVID-19 are a dry cough, feeling tired, fever and some people lose their sense of smell or taste. Others don't get any symptoms at all and mild symptoms can easily be mistaken for a common cold.

One of the more bizarre rumours I heard from a patient was that if you were able to hold your breath for more than ten seconds without feeling too uncomfortable, then you didn't have the infection. This is a grossly inaccurate way to diagnose or exclude COVID-19, but it may have convinced some people that they were virus-free before leaving the house and transmitting the infection to their close contacts.

My patient wasn't too happy to hear he still needed a test, even after showing me he could hold his breath for the allotted time.

CURES

Health authorities were at a loss as to what would actually help those who became infected, and answering 'I'm not sure,' doesn't build confidence. People want answers and they want them now.

Without any available treatments, people came up with their own solutions.

The false cures for COVID-19 that people were talking about included drinking scalding hot water, bleach or methanol. By July 2020, it was estimated that around the world approximately eight hundred people had died, nearly six thousand people had been hospitalised, and sixty had developed complete blindness after drinking methanol as a supposed cure for COVID-19.[9]

A much-touted preventative/cure in some parts of the community were drugs called hydroxychloroquine and azithromycin. This was followed by people recommending ivermectin and doxycycline. Strange combinations of drugs kept popping up and it was difficult to see where these suggestions were coming from.

I can understand why these drugs were tested on the virus in a lab setting – well-known medications are frequently repurposed. It makes sense to look for new ways to use old drugs. Drugs already approved for human use are known to be safe, or we know what we need to look out for and can monitor our patients for anticipated problems.

Hydroxychloroquine is used to decrease the body's overactive immune response in conditions like lupus and rheumatoid arthritis. SARS-CoV-2 is known to cause problems when the immune system becomes hyperactive, trying to eliminate the infection from the body. It's not a huge leap of logic to wonder if hydroxychloroquine would be helpful to dull the immune response, preventing the body from having an overzealous inflammatory reaction. At face value this theory seems plausible, but you still want to see it working in real life before offering it to patients. The medication comes with plenty of side effects, including the potential to cause a heart rhythm abnormality that can result in sudden death – not something you want to get wrong.

It can be helpful for people with autoimmune conditions as it decreases the inflammation in their joints, but we soon discovered that it may not be helpful for respiratory infections like COVID-19. Even if the drug works to inhibit viral replication in a lab, we might not find that it penetrates into the lung tissue where it needs to do its work.

Azithromycin is an antibiotic used to kill bacteria, but it is not known to have any particular antiviral action. This antibiotic is most often used for chest infections like pneumonia, for treating chlamydia and it is known to have a mild anti-inflammatory effect. It is usually safe in small doses, but prolonged courses of medication can cause side effects like drug-induced hepatitis and liver impairment.

In a lab setting, known drugs are tested to see if they can slow down or stop the growth of a particular bacteria or virus, then we use that information to direct further studies and see if it works in real life – outside of a petri dish. But it seems this step was being skipped.

Unfortunately some people seem to believe that if a drug has already gone through safety testing in humans and results in the lab look promising, then we should just go for it and start dishing it out. But it's a crucial step to check the drug works against the virus in vivo (in the body), and not just in vitro (in a test tube).

Throughout the early stages of the pandemic we had problems with people making incorrect assumptions. Even former US President Donald Trump spoke about the benefits of hydroxychloroquine. The idea snowballed, and in Australia Clive Palmer bought thirty million doses to distribute while

MP Craig Kelly shared the misinformation on his social media.[10]

Well-meaning doctors around the world began prescribing it to their patients as a preventative, which meant that some people who genuinely needed the drug to prevent their arthritis from flaring up missed out on their doses. Some of my patients with autoimmune conditions were forced to call pharmacy after pharmacy looking for a supply of their regular medication, petrified of missing doses and ending up debilitated with painful, inflamed joints.

Hydroxychloroquine as a preventative/cure was an idea that persisted well after health authorities around the world dismissed it as untrue. Some people felt it was their human right to be able to access a medication that was unproven to work against COVID-19.

This is a perfect example of how belief in a treatment, how we feel about it and how it is advertised to us as a solution, triggers our deeper emotional state and is able to surpass all intelligent discussion or debate.

By the end of 2020, two main treatments were found to benefit patients with severe COVID-19. Dexamethasone is a commonly used steroid that is found to be helpful for dulling down the immune system's overactive inflammatory response caused by the virus and lying patients on their stomach was another simple but effective measure to assist patients with their breathing while they were intubated in the intensive care unit.

Hydroxychloroquine became a political football and was eventually recommended by more politicians than physicians.

CONSPIRACY THEORIES

One of the strangest outcomes from the COVID-19 pandemic was the weird amalgamation of conspiracy theorists from all around the globe.

The anti-vaxxers found common ground with the anti-5G groups. Some claimed COVID-19 was a hoax and that this was all an incredible plot to control the population under a fascist regime. Others believed that COVID-19 was real, but thought it had been created by Bill Gates, who only wanted to use the COVID-19 vaccination to insert microchips into everyone. A few people even believed everything at once.

Then there was QAnon – a collective delusion of epic proportions that grew and grew throughout the pandemic.

For those of you who haven't heard of QAnon, it relates to the mysterious online presence of a man called 'Q' who claimed to be a high-level US Government official, rubbing shoulders with then President Donald Trump.

In a nutshell, the theory alleges that a secret 'deep state' group of cannibalistic paedophiles run the world and traffic children for sex, while drinking their blood to stay young. They also alleged that COVID-19 was a tool being used to control our lives.

When Melbourne's COVID-19 cases started to escalate in 2020 and the city went into lockdown, one of my patients told me it was all political camouflage, designed to keep everyone inside their homes in order to allow the US military to move in and free hundreds of thousands of sex-trafficked children from underground tunnels beneath the streets of Melbourne.

It might seem ridiculous, but mass delusions like these can have an impact on the effectiveness of public health policy.

In the US, QAnon had millions of online followers, and the number in Australia was estimated to be in the thousands. Many of the hard right extremists who stormed the US Capitol in January of 2021 wore clothing emblazoned with QAnon logos and believed they were doing their part to overthrow the 'deep state'.

Attempting to make sense from chaos is human nature – we constantly look for patterns and try to match everything up into a seamless narrative. Many people who were isolated at home with very little to do turned to the internet and social media to find answers, and the number of people lured down internet 'rabbit holes' substantially increased during the pandemic. False beliefs can spread quickly when they are shared online – well beyond their immediate circle of influence.

We live in an age where artificial intelligence and algorithms feed us our information diet.

Just like the food you eat, your online diet should be varied and nutritious, but the algorithms don't work like that.

If you watch a trashy piece of reality television on YouTube, the algorithm feeds you more of the same. Same goes for videos or articles about conspiracy theories, extremist views or bad health advice. These systems are designed to recommend content we will find intriguing, so that we keep reading and watching. Our social media feeds are filled with similar content, created to tantalise our brain and keep us hooked online.

The problem with these algorithms is that we end up seeing more and more of the same thing and end up with a blinkered view. We don't see all the possibilities of the world and the full flavour of everything contained within it; we just see more of the same view reinforced over and over again, even if that view is totally bananas.

So why am I worried about some strange conspiracy theories online? Well, I'm concerned about how this affects human behaviour.

When we're all trying to trudge our way through a COVID-19 pandemic and health authorities are telling us that we need to wear masks when we go outside, then we stand a chance of beating the virus. But people need to understand the science behind these decisions. They are simple enough concepts to grasp: if we wear a mask, we can stop ourselves from being exposed to a potentially deadly virus, and if we carry the virus inside our own lungs, we can prevent breathing that virus out onto other people.

Wearing a face mask or facial covering is a very small action that is also one of the most generous and respectful gifts you can give to others around you.

But if you believe the whole pandemic is a hoax, designed to control the population into compliant, sedated humanoids, then you're not going to bother wearing a mask. You can't catch a virus that doesn't exist, right?

The proliferation of problematic health advice is a serious issue that needs to be addressed in all aspects of society – it's just never been more apparent than during the COVID-19 pandemic.

CHAPTER 16

FIXING THE FUTURE

At the end of the day it's important to understand that being fed the wrong information can negatively impact a person's life – my own experiences are good examples of this.

Even when I knew I was gay, I struggled to come to terms with it because I was fed false information. From a young age I was taught that being gay was wrong and when I finally came out, I was told that I was broken and needed to be fixed. I was encouraged to cure my 'same-sex attraction disorder' by attending therapy, but I eventually discovered that you can't fix what isn't broken. The whole process was extremely distressing and prevented me from moving forward in life.

Similarly, when I felt fatigued but couldn't find a reason to explain it, I was again fed false information. I was told that I lacked vitamins, my adrenals were fatigued and I was possessed by demons. I pursued all kinds of unusual therapies, but none of them helped. Everything I went through was only a distraction until I finally found the answer in modern medicine.

Even after being diagnosed with narcolepsy and told that my brain didn't produce enough orexin – a wakefulness hormone – I was still fed false information. Dr Google advised me that I'd sleep much better if I kept the window open and placed my feet outside the bedsheets, but this only made me wake up during the night with frosty feet. A friendly naturopath told me to avoid fatty meals during the day because they would make me sleepy, but I'd doze off with or without a spaghetti carbonara under my belt. The only solution I have found came from following my sleep physician's advice.

Fake medicine is harmful. It provides us with the wrong diagnosis, offers us the wrong treatment, and distracts us from getting real medical help – but it's acceptable in supermarkets, health food stores, pharmacies and even medical clinics. Too often we turn a blind eye to it and allow other people to make mistakes instead of looking out for each other.

Wouldn't it be incredible to live in a society where fake medicine wasn't sold on every street corner? A world where you and your loved ones approached health care with a critical mind and a sceptical eye?

So, what can we do to rise up and fight fake medicine?

●

A number of years ago I was asked to appear on a television talk show to discuss the importance of getting the influenza jab in the lead-up to winter. This is something I'm usually happy to do – it's important to ensure appropriate information is being broadcast about such health topics – however, I declined the opportunity when I found out I would be expected to engage in a live debate with an anti-vaxxer.

Vaccinations aren't up for debate – as I've mentioned in this book, overwhelming scientific evidence has proven again and again that immunisations protect us from infectious diseases and are extremely well tolerated. Debating the benefits of vaccination is like debating the benefits of wearing a seatbelt.

Providing an anti-vaccination advocate the opportunity to speak beside a qualified doctor gives them credibility they don't deserve. I discussed this with the producers and explained why going ahead with the segment would be irresponsible.

Unfortunately, they didn't heed my advice, and the segment went to air with another medical professional in my place.

As I predicted, the anti-vaxxer hijacked the conversation by confidently making outlandish and untrue statements. They were able to use this national platform to share their beliefs and spoke for the majority of the five-minute health segment. The doctor representing the side of science couldn't possibly have rebutted all the ridiculous claims being made in the allotted time – the whole exercise was a predictable disaster.

This is just one example of the ongoing battle we face against fake medicine.

If you're keen to join me on the side of science and reason, then it's important to learn some of the tactics used against us. Let's start with a forensic deconstruction of this debating debacle.

FALSE BALANCE

This seemingly innocent debate only served to orchestrate false balance, where two unequal opponents are pitted against each other but presented as equals. It signals to the audience watching at home that both points of view are equally valid – all for the sake of creating argumentative fireworks on television.

However, the views are not equally valid. One is backed up by evidence, science and a medical degree – the other by discredited practitioners, retracted research and people who educated themselves by watching anti-vaccination propaganda videos on YouTube.

False balance essentially places one expert in their field against a charismatic idiot. It might be entertaining viewing, but it can easily seed doubt, undermine public health messages and ultimately discourage parents from vaccinating their children.[1]

Health experts dedicated to the fight against fake medicine need to refuse debating people with fringe views. Identifying where false balance may occur and preventing it from happening in the first place are the best things we can do.

Fortunately, many Australian media organisations have started taking steps to address the issue, altering their broadcasting policies in light of the potential damage false balance can cause. It's now extremely rare for anti-vaxxers or climate change deniers to be given airtime on television or radio. It still occasionally happens, and when it does, it's important to tell media organisations loudly and clearly that they are letting their audience down.

It's relatively easy to spot false balance if you're keeping an eye out for it – just pay attention to the credentials of the experts providing their opinions. A public health physician shouldn't debate a clairvoyant, climate scientists shouldn't compete with climate change deniers, and oncologists shouldn't be on the same panel as someone who believes they can cure cancer with prayer and a healthy diet.

GISH GALLOP

False balance wasn't the only issue my colleague encountered – the second problem they needed to face was the anti-vaxxer's 'Gish gallop'.

American anthropologist Eugenie Scott named this technique after Duane Gish, a creationist known to throw down a large number of false claims, half-truths, misrepresentations and twisted facts, all within a small amount of time at the start of a debate. The sheer number of false statements he was able to deliver overwhelmed his opponent.

It's easy to spit out a series of 'alternative facts' in rapid succession, but it takes time and effort to refute them. When a stack of misinformation is suddenly dropped in your lap, you simply don't have enough time to individually address, dismantle and debunk these incorrect statements during a five-minute television segment. If you are seen to struggle, the audience can interpret this as a sign of uncertainty.

Attempting to rebut every component of a Gish gallop is honourable, but it's disheartening when you invariably run out of time. This destructive debating technique is designed to derail the whole process of respectful discussion – and this is what happened to my colleague on the panel show.

This tactic isn't just limited to television studios – it's commonly used by relatives, so listen out for it during spirited political discussions at family gatherings.

In the end, there's no effective way to deal with a Gish galloper's verbal barrage. Rather than attempting to address all their arguments, you're better off pointing out the tactic to your audience and explaining that it's impossible to rebuke everything in the time available. Follow this up with a general statement to acknowledge and summarise your opponent's concerns and then continue with your own factual talking points. This brings the discussion back on track and prevents you and your audience from being distracted by the Gish gallop.

'JUST ASKING QUESTIONS'

Many fake medicine advocates claim that they are 'just asking questions' while they sow seeds of doubt. Like a solitary cough on a crowded bus, it takes little effort but makes everyone feel uneasy.

If fluoride is so safe and effective, why do we only put small amounts in our water?'

'If 5G doesn't cause COVID, *why was it being rolled out just as the pandemic began?'*

'I'm not saying the prime minister is a reptilian overlord, but when was the last time you saw them blink?'

This debating technique (sometimes abbreviated to 'JAQing off') allows people to casually insert their own extravagant musings, conspiracy theories and wild accusations into the conversation by framing statements as questions.

JAQing off is a great time-waster because the person asking questions is not looking for answers. The person who is *just asking questions* might think they are on the verge of unveiling a grand conspiracy, but may not realise that their questions only highlight their profound misunderstanding of a complex topic.

When you're battling fake medicine, feel free to answer questions grounded in reality – especially when you believe your answers will be taken seriously – but don't feel pressured to dignify disingenuous questions with a response. Some people are only out there to cause trouble.

REPETITION

Repeating the same incorrect statement over and over again won't make it come true, but after it has been said enough times some people might start believing it.

Donald Trump used a repetition technique throughout his presidency, especially during the COVID-19 pandemic. In 2020 he reassured the media at least thirty-eight times that the virus was just going to disappear – even in the face of escalating cases and overflowing hospitals.[2] While his original intention may have been to prevent panic and calm his followers, this repetition of misinformation undermined public health efforts and discouraged others from taking the outbreak seriously.

Familiarity and repetition will eat away at you slowly. They are able to cast doubt and gaslight you into agreement.

It's frustrating to see fake medicine memes repeatedly appear online, but it's even worse when you find out your sister is going to bed with onions in her socks. Encourage your family and friends to stop sharing incorrect information and ask them to fight fake medicine by thinking a little more critically.

MISREPRESENTATION

We like to trust in science and it would be great if we could believe that every study is accurate and truthful, but it's not that simple. You need to be aware that the conclusions from research papers are occasionally misrepresented, either by accident or on purpose. It's possible for the original data to be altered or corrupted, and statistical calculations can be manipulated or massaged, while the conclusion may be misinterpreted or politicised into a misrepresentation of true events.

Under normal circumstances there's a system in place where scientific studies are peer reviewed before results are released to the public. Peer-reviewed research means that other scientists have assessed the study by examining the raw data, double-checked the calculations and agree with the author's conclusion. We can be more confident that the results are accurate, trustworthy and meaningful after they've been examined by a team of pedantic professors.

But over the COVID-19 pandemic, we've been living through extenuating circumstances. In our rush to share valuable information, media releases and 'pre-print' research (before peer review) have made it into the public sphere without receiving the usual oversight. It's fantastic when the results are accurate because lifesaving information is able to get out there quickly, but a number of low-quality studies have slipped through the net.

Once fake medicine is released it's very difficult to put it all back in the retraction bin. Even after a study has been disproven, false information continues to be regurgitated online.

Journalists and science communicators act as translators for the public, relaying information from medical journals and interpreting research papers into easy-to-understand language. But people reporting the news are under great pressure during a crisis and may need to rely on media releases or pre-prints. This makes it even more important for you to take notice of where your information is coming from and the likely quality of that information.

TROLLING

Anyone approaching the front line to fight fake medicine needs to know about trolls. These mischievous creatures roam the internet looking for people to provoke. They intentionally cause trouble for their own personal amusement or act on behalf of an underlying agenda. The most important advice for dealing with a troll is not to lose your temper. They know how to get under your skin and are keen to incite anger and create chaos.

Civilised debate or dignified discussion are never on the cards as trolls will attempt to distract from and deflect the conversation at every opportunity. They are divisive and make inflammatory statements to polarise their audience.

Trolling is a blood sport for some people. Behind the scenes, a troll may thoroughly research their target, find out their personal history, harass them at their workplace, and return to deliver a scathing personal attack in order to discredit them. In some cases multiple social media accounts are used, either by a group of trolls deciding to pick on the same person or one person operating a number of different accounts.

Stolen identities may be used to impersonate or parody the troll's targets, while masquerading as a figure of authority is another way to influence others. Trolls have been known to invent conspiracy theories to push alternative agendas and nurture distrust. More elaborate trolls will even create pretend news organisations in order to distribute fake articles or propaganda. Understanding these practices is imperative, so you can recognise when they occur and hopefully sidestep some stress. Online, everything is not always what it seems.

●

We've discussed some of the common tricks and techniques used to manipulate others – and how to selectively use some of those tricks yourself – but now we need to look at the bigger picture. When misinformation is already a major problem and we expect it to get worse, what can you do to fix it?

BE PART OF THE SOLUTION

Fake medicine turns up uninvited on your television screen, social media feed, favourite podcast – it even sneaks into that kindly advice from your mum. But we all need to take responsibility and stop it impacting on our lives.

It's easy to click quick and ask questions later, but before you know it you've spread misinformation all over your social network – so one of the most important things you can do is to simply take a breath before reposting or retweeting.

You are the one who has curated your own social media network and it's your responsibility to make sure the information you share is trustworthy.

Imagine inviting all your friends around to your house for a roast dinner. You remove the chicken from your oven and begin to serve it around the table, but you haven't checked to see if it's fully cooked. Some of your friends trust you and start eating raw chicken even though it tastes a bit funny. Others politely ask why it's a little bit pink, while a few of your guests decide to just eat the vegetables. Dishing out misinformation is like serving up an uncooked chook – not all of your guests will be affected, but there's a real chance some of them could end up in hospital.

Misinformation can kill, so remember to slice into the centre of your facts to see if they are fully cooked before passing them on.

When your information seems a bit pinkish, go back to the original source and work out who wrote the article and who they interviewed, and check if it is from a website you trust.

It's also important to remember that someone will always be wrong on the internet so choose your battles wisely. When you do decide to lay down your gauntlet and engage online, keep in mind the goal is to make friends and win converts, not to destroy them. Be kind.

It's frustrating to see someone repeatedly post misinformed messages about Bill Gates injecting people with microchips, but it's even worse when it's your mum.

Fighting fake medicine can be much more difficult when you're dealing with family – the stakes are higher and they know how to push your buttons. It can take years of chipping away before you're able to change someone else's mind. It's easy to feel like you're wasting your time when your family don't seem to listen and won't acknowledge your politely worded feedback – but they are still family. You may never win them over, but the best weapons in your arsenal are patience, repetition, persistence, kindness and repetition.

There's no guarantee that your parents will stop protesting against fluoride or 5G, but there's always a chance your intervention might pay off – eventually.

PREBUNKING AND DEBUNKING

When you encounter misinformation in the heat of battle, the best tactic is to debunk. This involves explaining the science, revealing the truth and exposing nonsense – but how do you debunk?

I generally give online influencers a wide berth, but when it comes to countering misinformation, I find they are an odd source of inspiration. Even when their health advice is deplorable, it's hard to hate them – they are so loveable, positive and engaging. They know their target demographic and use language that is appropriate and easily understood. Influencers keep the conversation light, entertaining, informative and interesting.

In comparison, scientists aren't known to attract a massive online following but are more typically seen to be timid, socially awkward and intellectually bewildering. Academics may be experts in their field, but it takes a different set of skills to explain to the public what you're actually doing in the lab. Scientists need to learn from influencers' techniques if we want to get our messages across.

Good debunking involves getting to the point quickly. Keep your message simple, clear and concise. Break your information down into bite-sized pieces. Consider your audience and use words and analogies they will be able to understand.

But even before debunking, there's opportunity for prebunking – informing, explaining and educating people about all the different types of fake medicine before they encounter them in real life.

A great example of a prebunking initiative is being carried out in Finland. In 2014 the Finnish Government identified a growing problem with misinformation and announced a nationwide plan to provide their entire population with training in critical thinking. A new curriculum was rolled out across the country and Finnish citizens of all ages are now being taught how to spot fake news and think more clearly in an attempt to prevent propaganda, rumours or hoaxes from influencing their decisions.[3]

This education program wasn't designed to tell people *what* to think, instead the curriculum was created to teach people *how to think*, and to provide the nation with the cognitive tools to critically critique information presented in the media or online. Ultimately it aims to decrease the chance of being tricked.

Finland is now leading the fight in the battle against fake news.

And they're starting young. Even primary school children are learning how to assess information online. Everyone is taught how to differentiate advertising from journalism, how to recognise when an author is presenting biased information, and how to distinguish when a publisher might have an ulterior motive. Kids are being taught not to rely solely on sites like Wikipedia and are trained to check multiple sources before accepting any information as fact.[4]

Finnish citizens are exposed to different types of misinformation, which means that when they encounter dubious advice they are able to quickly identify it, avoid it and warn others about it. This essentially immunises their population against fake news. We should be learning from Finland's success and working to protect our own people from harm.

Thinking critically takes practice and the sooner we are taught to ground ourselves in science, the more successful our thinking will be as adults.

Immunise yourself and your loved ones against misinformation and join the fight to limit the spread of fake medicine.

THANK YOU

Massive thanks goes to Jamie Cummins for inspiring and encouraging me throughout this entire process. Thanks to Ted, Tracey, Josh, Sam, James and Humphrey for putting up with me hibernating for months. Thank you to John and Wendy for your unwavering support. Thank you to Dean, Anna and Isabella for welcoming me into your home and giving me space to write over a very strange COVID-19 festive season.

Thanks to Robert, Nita, Joanna, Claire, Scott, Joyce, Richard, Robert and Edna for providing me with the memories and material to create this book. Thanks to Caleb, Daniel, Riley, Conor and Bronte for providing me with the motivation to strengthen the critical thinking of generations to come.

Thanks to Eryn, Chloe, Harlow and Dexter for your thoughtfulness, kindness and pats.

The team at Hachette has been incredibly supportive, with Louise Adler as publisher to spur me on, Sophie Mayfield as a very understanding editor, Deonie Fiford as an extremely talented copy-editor, as well as Jenny Topham, Isabella Lloyd, Tessa Connelly and Christa Moffitt.

Trish Hann has been far too kind and read far too many versions of this book while still appearing sane. Thank you to Gideon Meyerowitz-Katz, Jessica Singer, Martin Hadley, Tim Mendham, Richard Saunders, Rachael Dunlop, Eran Segev, Lara Benham and Joshua Godbee for your dedication and valuable insights. Thank you to the Gaggle, Ashley Robison, Daniel Lang, Thomas Worrell, Tomas Warden, David MacNeil, Daniel de Moor, Matthew Langmaid, Nathan Beencke, Gareth Williams and Katie Dillon for your tolerance and assistance. Thank you to my evidence-based colleagues at East Sydney Doctors and to my patients for your inspiration and understanding.

Thank you to the many other special people who helped make this book a reality, including Ginni Mansberg, Daniel Rubinstein, Helen Schultz, Melanie Tait, Ginger Gorman, Julia Baird, Rick Morton, Stan Grant, Shannon Molloy, Rob Battisti, Cain Cooper, Jun Yang, Linda Cumines, Susie Burrell, Darren Saunders, Nicole Rogerson, Julie Leask, Peter Ebeling, Ian Musgrave, Mandy-Lee Noble, Daya Sharma, Matt Hopcraft, Ben Goldacre, Cara Santa Maria, Ken Harvey, John Skerritt, Nick Toscano, Beau Donelly, Stephanie Alice Baker, Chris Rojek, Nikki Stamp, Tim Minchin, Josh Thomas, Amy Remeikis, Todd Abbott, Ross Scheepers, Siobhan Hammer, Dean Webber, Reuben Cheok, Katrina Agnew, Trent Hessell, Amy Hessell, Theodore Dimaras, Lina Dimitropoulos, Vyom Sharma, Mike Todorovic, Robert Page and Vincent Cornelisse.

ENDNOTES

CHAPTER 2: ROOT CAUSE

1

R Baillie, 'Christian programs attempting to convert homosexuals
continue in Australia', *ABC News*, 30 July 2013, accessed 21 January
2021. https://www.abc.net.au/news/2013-07-30/christian-ex-gay-
conversion-programs-continue-in-australia/4854580

M Lallo, 'Ministries preying on gay shame', *The Age*, 8 April 2012,
accessed 21 January 2021. https://www.theage.com.au/national/
victoria/ministries-preying-on-gay-shame-20120407-1wif0.html

2

Royal College of Psychiatrists, 'Royal College of Psychiatrists' statement
on sexual orientation', Royal College of Psychiatrists, April
2014, accessed 21 January 2021. https://www.rcpsych.ac.uk/pdf/
PS02_2014.pdf

3

I Bieber, C R Herron, D Johnston, R Spitzer, 'The issue is subtle, the
debate still on', *The New York Times*, 23 December 1973. Accessed
21 January 2021. https://www.nytimes.com/1973/12/23/archives/the-
issue-is-subtle-the-debate-still-on-the-apa-ruling-on.html

American Psychiatric Association, *Diagnostic and Statistical Manual of
Mental Disorders* (2nd edition, revised), Washington DC, 1974

J Drescher, 'Out of DSM: Depathologizing homosexuality', *Behavioral Sciences*, 2015, 5(4): 565–575. https://doi.org/10.3390/bs5040565

CHAPTER 3: DR GOOGLE

1

M Murphy, 'Dr Google will see you now: Search giant wants to cash in on your medical queries', *The Telegraph*, 10 March 2019, accessed 21 January 2021. https://www.telegraph.co.uk/technology/2019/03/10/google-sifting-one-billion-health-questions-day/

2

M Hill, B Mills, M Sim, 'The quality of diagnosis and triage advice provided by free online symptom checkers and apps in Australia', *The Medical Journal of Australia*, 2020, 212(11), 514–519. https://doi.org/10.5694/mja2.50600

CHAPTER 4: THE WHOLE PANTRY OF LIES

1

P Barry, 'How the media fell for Belle', *Media Watch*, ABC, 16 March 2015, accessed 21 January 2021. https://www.abc.net.au/mediawatch/episodes/how-the-media-fell-for-belle/9973312

B Donelly, N Toscano, 'Refund calls over "cancer survivor" Belle Gibson's book and app sales', *The Sydney Morning Herald,* 11 March 2015, accessed 21 January 2021. https://www.smh.com.au/technology/refund-calls-over-cancer-survivor-belle-gibsons-book-and-app-sales-20150311-141by8.html

M Friedman, 'Twentysomething Instagram celebrity accused of faking her cancer diagnosis', *Cosmopolitan*, 13 March 2015, accessed 21 January 2021. https://www.cosmopolitan.com/lifestyle/news/a37731/belle-gibson-the-whole-pantry-cancer-diagnosis/

V Lawrence, 'What we know about Belle Gibson', *Elle Australia*, 13 March 2015, accessed 21 January 2021. https://www.elle.com.au/news/what-we-know-about-belle-gibson-5919

2

B Donelly, N Toscano, 'Publisher Penguin pulls Belle Gibson cook book The Whole Pantry', *The Sydney Morning Herald*, 16 March 2015, accessed 21 January 2021. https://www.smh.com.au/national/publisher-penguin-pulls-belle-gibson-cook-book-the-whole-pantry-20150316-1m0dsc.html

M Smith, 'The "hole" in the pantry story: should Penguin have validated Belle Gibson's cancer claims?', *The Conversation*, 16 March 2015, accessed 21 January 2021. https://theconversation.com/the-hole-in-the-pantry-story-should-penguin-have-validated-belle-gibsons-cancer-claims-38843

3

B Donelly, N Toscano, 'Charity money promised by "inspirational" health app developer Belle Gibson not handed over', *The Sydney Morning Herald*, 8 March 2015, accessed 21 January 2021. https://www.smh.com.au/technology/charity-money-promised-by-inspirational-health-app-developer-belle-gibson-not-handed-over-20150306-13xgqk.html

4

B Donelly, N Toscano, 'Backlash over app developer Belle Gibson's missing charity money', *The Sydney Morning Herald*, 9 March 2015, accessed 21 January 2021. https://www.smh.com.au/technology/backlash-over-app-developer-belle-gibsons-missing-charity-money-20150309-13yzd4.html

5

C Weaver, 'Belle Gibson: my lifelong struggle with the truth', *The Australian Women's Weekly*, 23 April 2015, accessed 21 January 2021. nowtolove.co.nz/news/real-life/belle-gibson-my-lifelong-struggle-with-the-truth-6860/

6

Federal Court of Australia, *Director of Consumer Affairs Victoria v Gibson (No 2)* 2017 FCA 366, 7 April 2017. https://www.consumer.vic.gov.au/latest-news/annabelle-gibson-and-inkerman-road-nominees-pty-ltd-court-action

7

'Belle Gibson's home in Melbourne raided over $500,000 in unpaid fines', *ABC News*, 22 January 2020, accessed 21 January 2021. https://www.abc.net.au/news/2020-01-22/belle-gibson-raided-over-500k-in-unpaid-fines/11890094

8

'Belle Gibson, disgraced "wellness" advocate, facing legal action over cancer claims', *ABC News*, 6 May 2016, accessed 21 January 2021. https://www.abc.net.au/news/2016-05-06/belle-gibson-legal-action-to-be-taken-against-wellness-advocate/7390612

9

L Burke, '"They are all complicit": Cancer researcher Dr Darren Saunders slams Belle Gibson's "enablers"', news.com.au, 23 April 2015, accessed 21 January 2021. https://www.news.com.au/lifestyle/health/health-problems/they-are-all-complicit-cancer-researcher-dr-darren-saunders-slams-belle-gibsons-enablers/news-story/f53198d4e359b74609134a44d7a54a5f

CHAPTER 5: THE POWER OF INFLUENCERS

1

S Stevenson, 'How I healed myself naturally: cervical dysplasia CIN 3 (high grade)', Sarah's Day, 25 July 2018, accessed 21 January 2021. https://www. youtube.com/watch?v=tsIBcEzlb9Y

2

M Andrews, 'The dark side of Instagram influencers', news.com.au, 3 August 2018, accessed 21 January 2021. https://www.news.com.au/lifestyle/real-life/news-life/the-dark-side-of-instagram-influencers/news-story/9538cd51f9f0a8c45dca4da42080967e

3

S Stevenson, 'How I healed myself naturally: cervical dysplasia CIN 3 (high grade)', Sarah's Day, 25 July 2018, accessed 21 January 2021. https://www. youtube.com/watch?v=tsIBcEzlb9Y

4

S Baker, C Rojek, *Lifestyle Gurus: Constructing authority and influence online*, Polity Press, Cambridge, UK, 2019, pp.6–7.

5

Hootsuite & We Are Social, 'Digital 2020: Australia', Datareportal, 13 February 2020, accessed 21 January 2021. https://datareportal. com/reports/digital-2020-australia

6

N Stamp, *Pretty Unhealthy: Why our obsession with looking healthy is making us sick*, Murdoch Books, Sydney, 2019.

7

J Ainscough, 'No ill will', *ABC News*, 7 April 2010, accessed 21 January 2021. https://www.abc.net.au/news/2010-04-07/33482

8

J Ainscough, 'No ill will', *ABC News*, 7 April 2010, accessed 21 January 2021. https://www.abc.net.au/news/2010-04-07/33482

'Questionable methods of cancer management: "Nutritional" therapies', *CA: A cancer journal for clinicians*, 43(5), 309–319. https://doi. org/10.3322/canjclin.43.5.309

9

S Baker, C Rojek, *Lifestyle Gurus: Constructing authority and influence online*, Polity Press, Cambridge, UK, 2019.

10

D Saunders, 'Stealing from the wellness gurus', *Ockham's Razor with Robyn Williams*, ABC Radio, 16 September 2018, accessed 21 January 2021. https://www.abc.net.au/radionational/ programs/ockhamsrazor/stealing-from-wellness-gurus-darren-saunders/10243090

CHAPTER 6: THOUSANDS OF YEARS

1

E Crighton, ML Coghlan, R Farrington, CL Hoban, MWP Power, C Nash, I Mullaney, RW Byard, R Trengove, IF Musgrave, M Bunce, G Maker, 'Toxicological screening and DNA sequencing detects contamination and adulteration in regulated herbal medicines and supplements for diet, weight loss and cardiovascular health', *Journal of Pharmaceutical and Biomedical Analysis*, 2019, 176, 112834. https://doi.org/10.1016/j.jpba.2019.112834

2

M Standaert, '"This makes Chinese medicine look bad": TCM supporters condemn illegal wildlife trade', *The Guardian*, 26 May 2020, accessed 21 January 2021. https://www.theguardian.com/environment/2020/may/26/its-against-nature-illegal-wildlife-trade-casts-shadow-over-traditional-chinese-medicine-aoe

3

Australian Acupuncture & Chinese Medicine Association, 'Acupuncture & Chinese Medicine', 2021, accessed 21 January 2021. https://www.acupuncture.org.au/acupuncture-chinese-medicine/acupuncture

4

M Johnson, C Paley 'Acupuncture for the relief of chronic pain: A synthesis of systematic reviews', *Medicina*, 2019, 56(1), 6. https://doi.org/10.3390/medicina56010006

5

D Godson, J Wardle, 'Accuracy and precision in acupuncture point location: A critical systematic review', *Journal of Acupuncture and Meridian Studies*, 2019, 12 (2), 52–66. https://doi.org/10.1016/j.jams.2018.10.009

6

MS Lee, J Kang, E Ernst, 'Does moxibustion work? An overview of systematic reviews', *BMC Res Notes*, 5 November 2010, 3, 284. https://doi.org/10.1186/1756-0500-3-284

7

ME Coyle, CA Smith, B Peat, 'Cephalic version by moxibustion for breech presentation', *The Cochrane database of systematic reviews*, 16 May 2012, (5), accessed 15 February 2021. https://doi.org/10.1002/14651858.CD003928.pub3

8

D Charles, T Hudgins, J MacNaughton, E Newman, J Tan, M Wigger, 'A systematic review of manual therapy techniques, dry cupping and dry needling in the reduction of myofascial pain and myofascial trigger points', *Journal of Bodywork and Movement Therapies*, 2019, 23(3), 539–546. https://doi.org/10.1016/j.jbmt.2019.04.001

MS Lee, JI Kim, E Ernst, 'Is cupping an effective treatment? An overview of systematic reviews', *Journal of Acupuncture and Meridian Studies*, 2011, 4(1), 1–4. https://doi.org/10.1016/S2005-2901(11)60001-0

9

Harvard Health Publishing, Harvard Medical School, 'The health benefits of tai chi', *Harvard Women's Health Watch*, 20 August 2019, accessed 21 January 2021. https://www.health.harvard.edu/staying-healthy/the-health-benefits-of-tai-chi

CHAPTER 7: TWEAKING, BOOSTING AND RATTLING

1

National Institute for Health and Care Excellence (NICE), 'Chronic fatigue syndrome/myalgic encephalomyelitis (or encephalopathy): diagnosis and management', 22 August 2007. https://www.nice.org.uk/guidance/cg53/chapter/1-Guidance#general-management-strategies-after-diagnosis.
Note that this is reiterated in the draft for the final guidelines, set to be published in April 2021.

U.S. ME/CFS Clinician Coalition, 'Diagnosing and treating myalgic encephalomyelitis/chronic fatigue syndrome (ME/CFS)', July 2020, Version 2. https://www.omf.ngo/2019/09/01/new-guidelines-for-diagnosing-and-treating-me-cfs/

2

S Spedding, 'Vitamins are more funky than Casimir thought', *Australasian Medical Journal*, 2013, 6(2), 104–106.

3

Roy Morgan, 'Over 8.3 million Australians buy vitamins, minerals and supplements', 26 April 2019, accessed 21 January 2021. http://www.roymorgan.com/findings/7956-australian-vitamin-market-december-2018-201904260734

4

SBS, 'Vitamins & Supplements', *SBS Insight*, 2019, 12 March 2019. https://www.sbs.com.au/ondemand/video/1448561731545

5

SBS, 'Vitamins & Supplements', *SBS Insight*, 2019, 12 March 2019.
   https://www.sbs.com.au/ondemand/video/1448561731545

6

SBS, 'Vitamins & Supplements', *SBS Insight*, 2019, 12 March 2019.
   https://www.sbs.com.au/ondemand/video/1448561731545

K Harvey, 'TGA endorses pseudoscience for complementary
   meds', *Australasian Science*, 2017, 38(5), 44. http://www.
   australasianscience.com.au/article/issue-sepoct-2017/tga-endorses-
   pseudoscience-complementary-meds.html

7

SBS, 'Vitamins & Supplements', *SBS Insight*, 2019, 12 March 2019.
   https://www.sbs.com.au/ondemand/video/1448561731545

8

Complementary Medicines Australia, 'Australia's Complementary
   Medicines Industry Audit & Trends 2020', 2020, accessed 21 January
   2021. https://www.cmaustralia.org.au/resources/CMA-industry-
   presentation-2020.pdf

9

A Rohner, K Ried, IA Sobenin, HC Bucher, AJ Nordmann, 'A systematic
   review and metaanalysis on the effects of garlic preparations on
   blood pressure in individuals with hypertension', *American Journal
   of Hypertension*, 2015, 28(3), 414–423. https://doi.org/10.1093/ajh/
   hpu165

10

N Namazi, K Khodamoradi, SP Khamechi, J Heshmati, MH Ayati,
   B Larijani, 'The impact of cinnamon on anthropometric indices
   and glycemic status in patients with type 2 diabetes: A systematic
   review and meta-analysis of clinical trials', *Complementary
   Therapies in Medicine*, 2019, 43, 92–101. https://doi.org/10.1016/j.
   ctim.2019.01.002

11

PA Pinzón-Arango, Y Liu, TA Camesano, 'Role of cranberry on bacterial
   adhesion forces and implications for *Escherichia coli*–uroepithelial

cell attachment', *Journal of Medicinal Food*, 2009, 12(2), 259–270. https://doi.org/10.1089/jmf.2008.0196

12

RG Jepson, G Williams, JC Craig, 'Cranberries for preventing urinary tract infections', *Cochrane Database of Systematic Reviews*, 2012, 10, CD001321. https://doi.org/10.1002/14651858.CD001321.pub5

13

KC Maki, KL Kaspar, C Khoo, LH Derrig, AL Schild, K Gupta, 'Consumption of a cranberry juice beverage lowered the number of clinical urinary tract infection episodes in women with a recent history of urinary tract infection', *The American Journal of Clinical Nutrition*, 2016, 103(6), 1434–1442. https://doi.org/10.3945/ajcn.116.130542

14

M Juthani-Mehta, PH Van Ness, L Bianco, et al, 'Effect of cranberry capsules on bacteriuria plus pyuria among older women in nursing homes: A randomized clinical trial', *The Journal of the American Medical Association*, 2016, 316(18), 1879–1887. doi:10.1001/jama.2016.16141

15

F Khorasani, H Aryan, A Sobhi, R Aryan, A Abavi-Sani, M Ghazanfarpour, M Saeidi, F Rajab Dizavandi, 'A systematic review of the efficacy of alternative medicine in the treatment of nausea and vomiting of pregnancy', *Journal of Obstetrics and Gynaecology*, 2020, 40(1), 10–19. https://doi.org/10.1080/01443615.2019.1587392

16

BB Albert, JGB Derraik, D Cameron-Smith, PL Hofman, S Tumanov, SG Villas-Boas, ML Garg, WS Cutfield, 'Fish oil supplements in New Zealand are highly oxidised and do not meet label content of n-3 PUFA', *Scientific Reports*, 2015, 5, 7928. https://doi.org/10.1038/srep07928

17

T Aung, J Halsey, D Kromhout, HC Gerstein, R Marchioli, et al, 'Associations of Omega-3 Fatty Acid Supplement Use With Cardiovascular Disease Risks: Meta-analysis of 10 Trials Involving

77 917 Individuals', *JAMA Cardiology*, 2018, 3(3), 225–234. https://doi.org/10.1001/jamacardio.2017.5205

18

Arthritis Australia, 'Arthritis Information Sheet', December 2007, accessed 21 January 2021. https://arthritisaustralia.com.au/wordpress/wp-content/uploads/2018/02/Fishoils.pdf

Arthritis Australia, 'Fish Oils', accessed 21 January 2021. https://arthritisaustralia.com.au/managing-arthritis/living-with-arthritis/complementary-treatments-and-therapies/fish-oils/

19

J Tomé-Carneiro, M Larrosa, A González-Sarrías, FA Tomás-Barberán, MT García-Conesa, JC Espín, 'Resveratrol and clinical trials: The crossroad from in vitro studies to human evidence', *Current Pharmaceutical Design*, 2013, 19(34), 6064–6093. https://doi.org/10.2174/13816128113199990407

JW Kim, DY Lee, BC Lee, MH Jung, H Kim, YS Choi, I-G Choi, 'Alcohol and cognition in the elderly: A review', *Psychiatry Investigation*, 2012, 9(1), 8–16. https://doi.org/10.4306/pi.2012.9.1.8

20

MM Jeyaraman, NSH Al-Yousif, A Singh Mann, VW Dolinsky, R Rabbani, R Zarychanski, AM Abou-Setta, 'Resveratrol for adults with type 2 diabetes mellitus', Cochrane Database of Systematic Reviews, 2020, 2, CD011919. https://doi.org//10.1002/14651858.CD011919.pub2

MM McDermott, C Leeuwenburgh, JM Guralnik, L Tian, R Sufit, L Zhao, MH Criqui, MR Kibbe, JH Stein, D Lloyd-Jones, SD Anton, TS Polonsky, Y Gao, R de Cabo, L Ferrucci, 'Effect of resveratrol on walking performance in older people with peripheral artery disease: The RESTORE randomized cinical trial', *Journal of the American Medical Association (JAMA) Cardiology*, 2(8), 902–907. https://doi.org/10.1001/jamacardio.2017.0538

A Soare, EP Weiss, JO Holloszy, L Fontana, 'Multiple dietary supplements do not affect metabolic and cardiovascular health', *Aging*, 2013, 6(2), 149–157. https://doi.org/10.18632/aging.100597

21

'Raw milk company Mountain View Farm defends product after 3yo's death', *ABC News*, 11 December 2014, accessed 21 January 2021. https://www.abc.net.au/news/2014-12-11/raw-milk-company-defends-product-after-3yos-death/5959246

R Lester, 'Unpasteurised milk health warning: 2 December 2014', Chief Health Officer, Department of Health and Human Services Victoria, 2 December 2014, accessed 21 January 2021. https://www2.health. vic.gov.au/about/news-and-events/healthalerts/advisory-2014-12-unpasteurised-milk-health-warning

CHAPTER 8: QUACKS

1

J Wardle, 'The Australian government review of natural therapies for private health insurance: What does it say and what does it mean?', *Advances in Integrative Medicine*, April 2016, 3(1), 3–10. https://doi. org/10.1016/j.aimed.2016.07.004

2

Cancer Research UK, 'Gerson therapy', 5 April 2019, accessed 21 January 2021. https://www.cancerresearchuk.org/about-cancer/cancer-in-general/treatment/complementary-alternative-therapies/individual-therapies/gerson

American Cancer Society, 'Unproven methods of cancer management: Gerson method', *CA: A Cancer Journal for Clinicians*, 1990, 40(4), 252–256. https://doi.org/10.3322/canjclin.40.4.252

American Cancer Society, 'Questionable methods of cancer management: "Nutritional" therapies', *CA: A Cancer Journal for Clinicians*, 1993, 43(5), 309–319. https://doi.org/10.3322/canjclin.43.5.309

3

Gerson Institute, 'The Gerson Therapy', 16 September 2011, accessed 21 January 2021. https://gerson.org/gerpress/the-gerson-therapy/

M Davey, 'Jessica Ainscough, Australia's "wellness warrior", dies of cancer aged 30', *The Guardian*, 1 March 2015, accessed 21 January 2021. https://www.theguardian.com/australia-news/2015/mar/01/jessica-ainscough-australia-wellness-warrior-dies-cancer-aged-30

4

'NHMRC statement: Statement on homeopathy', Australian Government
    National Health and Medical Research Council, March 2015,
    accessed 21 January 2021. https://www.nhmrc.gov.au/about-us/
    resources/homeopathy#block-views-block-file-attachments-content-
    block-1

5

NT Bateman, RM Leach, 'ABC of oxygen. Acute oxygen therapy', *The*
    British Medical Journal Clinical Research Edition, 1998, 317(7161),
    798–801. https://doi.org/10.1136/bmj.317.7161.798

6

E Ernst, 'Iridology: A systematic review', *Forschende*
    Komplementarmedizin, 1999, 6(1), 7–9. https://doi.
    org/10.1159/000021201

7

CJ Murphy, J Paul-Murphy, 'Iridology', *Journal of the American*
    Medical Association (JAMA) Ophthalmology, 2000, 118(8), 1140.
    https://jamanetwork.com/journals/jamaophthalmology/article-
    abstract/413509

8

E Ernst, P Posadzki, MS Lee, 'Reflexology: An update of a systematic
    review of randomised clinical trials', *Maturitas*, 2011, 68(2), 116–
    120. https://doi.org/10.1016/j.maturitas.2010.10.011

9

SM Rubinstein, A de Zoete, M van Middelkoop, WJJ Assendelft,
    MR de Boer, MW van Tulder, 'Benefits and harms of spinal
    manipulative therapy for the treatment of chronic low back pain:
    systematic review and meta-analysis of randomised controlled trials',
    The British Medical Journal Clinical Research Edition, 2019, 364,
    1689. https://doi.org/10.1136/bmj.l689

10

'Man "broke neck during chiropractor treatment" in York', *BBC News*,
    11 November 2019, accessed 21 January 2021. https://www.bbc.com/
    news/uk-england-york-north-yorkshire-50380928

11

RC Turner, BP Lucke-Wold, S Boo, CL Rosen, CL Sedney, 'The potential dangers of neck manipulation & risk for dissection and devastating stroke: An illustrative case & review of the literature', *Journal of Biomedical Research and Reviews*, 2018, 2(1), 10.15761/BRR.1000110. https://doi.org/10.15761/BRR.1000110

12

American Chiropractic Association, 'Origins and history of chiropractic care', 2021, accessed 21 January 2021. https://www.acatoday.org/About/History-of-Chiropractic

TJ Kaptchuk, DM Eisenberg, 'Chiropractic: Origins, controversies, and contributions', *Archives of Internal Medicine / Journal of the American Medical Association (JAMA)*, 1998, 158(20), 2215–2224. https://doi.org/10.1001/archinte.158.20.2215

13

DD Palmer, *Text-book of the Science, Art and Philosophy of Chiropractic*, Portland Printing House Company, Portland, Oregon, 1910.

14

E Ernst, A Gilbey, 'Chiropractic claims in the English-speaking world', *The New Zealand Medical Journal*, 2010, 123(1312), 36–44. https://pubmed.ncbi.nlm.nih.gov/20389316/

15

J Medew, 'Doctors at war with chiropractors over treatment of babies and children', *The Age*, 28 April 2016, accessed 21 January 2021. https://www.theage.com.au/healthcare/doctors-at-war-with-chiropractors-over-treatment-of-babies-and-children-20160428-gohlc9.html

R Spooner, 'Strict conditions slapped on chiropractor Dr Ian Rossborough', *The Age*, 9 June 2016, accessed 21 January 2021. https://www.theage.com.au/national/victoria/strict-conditions-slapped-on-chiropractor-dr-ian-rossborough-20160609-gpf299.html

R Sullivan, 'Chiropractor Dr Ian Rossborough defends cracking baby's back in awkward Studio 10 interview', news.com.au, 4 May 2016, accessed 21 January 2021. https://www.news.com.au/lifestyle/

parenting/babies/chiropractor-dr-ian-rossborough-defends-cracking-babys-back-in-awkward-studio-10-interview/news-story/92a6cb1906c97143a76dcfa2ce8d65f4

16

'Cranbourne chiropractor manipulates baby's spine in "deeply disturbing" video', *ABC News*, 20 February 2019, accessed 21 January 2021. https://www.abc.net.au/news/2019-02-20/chiropractor-baby-video-appalling-says-victorian-health-minister/10827976

17

Safer Care Victoria, 'Chiropractic spinal manipulation of children under 12', Safer Care Victoria, 24 October 2019, accessed 21 January 2021. https://www.bettersafercare.vic.gov.au/sites/default/files/2019-10/20191024-Final%20Chiropractic%20Spinal%20Manipulation.pdf

CHAPTER 10: SEXIST MEDICINE

1

'The heart attack gender gap: heart attacks strike men at younger ages than women. But survival rates are worse in women. Why?', *Harvard Heart Letter*, Harvard Medical School, April 2016, accessed 21 January 2021. https://www.health.harvard.edu/heart-health/the-heart-attack-gender-gap#:~:text=On%20average%2C%20a%20first%20heart,women%20as%20well%20as%20men

F Mauvais-Jarvis, NB Merz, PJ Barnes, RD Brinton, JJ Carrero, DL DeMeo, et al, 'Sex and gender: Modifiers of health, disease, and medicine', *The Lancet*, 2020, 396(10250), 565–582. https://doi.org/10.1016/S0140-6736(20)31561-0

LS Mehta, TM Beckie, HA DeVon, CL Grines, HM Krumholz, MN Johnson, KJ Lindley, V Vaccarino, TY Wang, KE Watson, NK Wenger, et al, 'Acute myocardial infarction in women: A scientific statement from the American Heart Association', *Circulation*, 2016, 133(9), 916–947. https://doi.org/10.1161/CIR.0000000000000351

2

J Billock, 'Pain bias: The health inequality rarely discussed', BBC Future, 22 May 2018, accessed 21 January 2021. https://www.bbc.com/

future/article/20180518-the-inequality-in-how-women-are-treated-for-pain

3

C Criado-Perez, 'The deadly truth about a world built for men – from stab vests to car crashes', *The Guardian,* 23 February 2019, accessed 21 January 2021. https://www.theguardian.com/lifeandstyle/2019/feb/23/truth-world-built-for-men-car-crashes

4

HE O'Connell, JM Hutson, CR Anderson, RJ Plenter, 'Anatomical relationship between urethra and clitoris', *The Journal of Urology*, 1998, 159(6), 1892–1897. https://doi.org/10.1016/SC02-5347(01)63188-4

HE O'Connell, JOL DeLancey, 'Clitoral anatomy in nulliparous, healthy, premenopausal volunteers using unenhanced magnetic resonance imaging', *The Journal of Urology*, 2005, 173(6), 2060–2063. https://doi.org/10.1097/01.ju.0000158446.21396.c0

C Wahlquist, 'The sole function of the clitoris is female orgasm. Is that why it's ignored by medical science?', *The Guardian*, 1 November 2020, accessed 21 January 2021. https://www.theguardian.com/lifeandstyle/2020/nov/01/the-sole-function-of-the-clitoris-is-female-orgasm-is-that-why-its-ignored-by-medical-science

5

HJ Teede, 'Advancing women in medical leadership', *The Medical Journal of Australia*, 2019, 211(9), 392–394. https://doi.org/10.5694/mja2.50287

6

X Lei, P Xu, B Cheng, 'Problems and solutions for platelet-rich plasma in facial rejuvenation: A systematic review', *Aesthetic Plastic Surgery*, 2019, 43(2), 457–469. https://doi.org/10.1007/s00266-018-1256-1

S Barr, 'Vampire facial: What is it and why is it so popular?', *The Independent*, 5 November 2020 (originally published in 2019), accessed 21 January 2021. https://www.independent.co.uk/life-style/fashion/vampire-facial-cost-benefits-what-is-it-kim-kardashian-beauty-treatment-a8232696.html

7

P Vazquez-Revuelta, R Madrigal-Burgaleta, 'Death due to Live Bee Acupuncture Apitherapy', *Journal of Investigational Allergonalology and Clinical Immunology*, 2018, 28(1), 45–46. https://doi. org/10.18176/jiaci.0202

8

J Belluz, 'Goop was fined $145,000 for its claims about jade eggs for vaginas. It's still selling them', Vox, 6 September 2018, accessed 21 January 2021. https://www.vox.com/2018/9/6/17826924/goop-yoni-egg-gwyneth-paltrow-settlement

9

SE Garcia, 'Goop agrees to pay $145,000 for "unsubstantiated" claims about vaginal eggs', *The New York Times*, 5 September 2018, accessed 21 January 2021. https://www.nytimes.com/2018/09/05/ business/goop-vaginal-egg-settlement.html

10

S Youn, 'Gwyneth Paltrow's goop settles vaginal eggs claims', (US) *ABC News*, 6 September 2018, accessed 21 January 2021. https:// abcnews.go.com/US/gwyneth-paltrows-goop-settles-vaginal-eggs-claims/story?id=57618571

CHAPTER 11: LOSING IT

1

Scamwatch, 'Report a scam', Australian Competition & Consumer Commission, accessed 21 January 2021. https://www.scamwatch.gov. au/report-a-scam

2

F Prior, M Workman, 'How TV's Dr Brad McKay became the face of an online keto pill scam', *ABC News*, 17 November 2020, accessed 21 January 2021. https://www.abc.net.au/news/2020-11-17/how-dr-brad-mckay-became-the-victim-of-online-scammers/12886458

3

KH Mikkelsen, T Seifert, NH Secher, T Grøndal, G van Hall, 'Systemic, cerebral and skeletal muscle ketone body and energy metabolism during acute hyper-D-β-hydroxybutyratemia in post-absorptive healthy males', *The Journal of Clinical Endocrinology and Metabolism*, 2015, 100(2), 636–643. https://doi.org/10.1210/jc.2014-2608

AKP Taggart, J Kero, X Gan, T-Q Cai, K Cheng, M Ippolito, N Ren, R Kaplan, K Wu, T-J Wu, L Jin, C Liaw, R Chen, J Richman, D Connolly, S Offermanns, SD Wright, MG Waters, '(d)-β-hydroxybutyrate inhibits adipocyte lipolysis via the nicotinic acid receptor PUMA-G', *Journal of Biological Chemistry*, 2005, 280(29), 26649–26652. https://doi.org/10.1074/jbc.C500213200

4

RJ Smith, C Bertilone, AG Robertson, 'Fulminant liver failure and transplantation after use of dietary supplements', *The Medical Journal of Australia*, 2016, 204(1), 30–32. https://doi.org/10.5694/mja15.00816

5

S Scott, A Branley, C Bembridge, 'Man given two weeks to live after taking popular weight-loss product purchased online', *ABC News*, 14 February 2016, accessed 21 January 2021. https://www.abc.net.au/news/2016-02-14/man-faced-death-after-taking-popular-weight-loss-product/7162378?nw=0

6

H Moskowitz, 'Bliss point: How food companies make us crave their products', retroreport.org, 3 January 2016, accessed 21 January 2021. https://www.retroreport.org/video/mini-doc/the-bliss-point/

7

Australian Government, 'Australia's health 2020: Overweight and obesity', Australian Institute of Health and Welfare, 23 July 2020, accessed 21 January 2021. https://www.aihw.gov.au/reports/australias-health/overweight-and-obesity

8

P Clifton, 'The science behind weight loss diets – A brief review', *Australian Family Physician*, 2006, 35(8), 580–582.

9

SD Anton, A Hida, K Heekin, K Sowalsky, C Karabetian, H Mutchie, C Leeuwenburgh, TM Manini, TE Barnett, 'Effects of popular diets without specific calorie targets on weight loss outcomes: Systematic review of findings from clinical trials', *Nutrients*, 2017, 9(8), 822. https://doi.org/10.3390/nu9080822

10

CE Kearns, LA Schmidt, SA Glantz, 'Sugar industry and coronary heart disease research: A historical analysis of internal industry documents', *Journal of the American Medical Association (JAMA) Internal Medicine*, 2016, 176(11), 1680–1685. https://doi.org/10.1001/jamainternmed.2016.5394

11

A Gupta, LG Smithers, A Braunack-Mayer, J Harford, 'How much free sugar do Australians consume? Findings from a national survey', *Australian and New Zealand Journal of Public Health*, 2018, 42(6), 533–540. https://doi.org/10.1111/1753-6405.12836

12

Q Yang, Z Zhang, EW Gregg, WD Flanders, R Merritt, FB Hu, 'Added sugar intake and cardiovascular diseases mortality among US adults', *Journal of the American Medical Association (JAMA) Internal Medicine*, 2014, 174(4), 516–524. https://doi.org/10.1001/jamainternmed.2013.13563

13

Dietitians Association of Australia, 'Aussies wasting time and money on pricey fad diets', 11 January 2017, accessed 21 January 2021. https://dietitiansaustralia.org.au/wp-content/uploads/2016/05/Aussies-wasting-time-and-money-on-pricey-fad-diets-FINAL.pdf

CHAPTER 13: ANTI-VAXXERS

1

FH Beard, J Leask, PB McIntyre, 'No Jab, No Pay and vaccine refusal in Australia: the jury is out', *The Medical Journal of Australia*, 2017, 206(9), 381–383. https://doi.org/10.5694/mja16.00944

2

J Medew, 'Anti-vaccination group encourages parents to join fake church', *The Sydney Morning Herald*, 27 January 2015, accessed 21

January 2021. https://www.smh.com.au/healthcare/antivaccination-group-encourages-parents-to-join-fake-church-20150127-12zcrc.html

A Wood, 'Anti-vaccine zealots form sham church', news.com.au, 30 May 2013, accessed 21 January 2021. https://www.news.com.au/lifestyle/health/anti-vaccine-zealots-form-sham-church/news-story/1da284692 59eeb56c33d3bf80b2dd684

3

F Chaib, H Hasan, 'New measles surveillance data for 2019', World Health Organization, 15 May 2019, accessed 21 January 2021. https://www.who.int/news/item/15-05-2019-new-measles-surveillance-data-for-2019

4

Pacific Beat, 'Samoan nurses jailed over deaths of two babies who were given incorrectly mixed vaccines', *ABC News*, 2 August 2019, accessed 21 January 2021. https://www.abc.net.au/news/2019-08-02/samoa-nurses-sentenced-manslaughter-infant-vaccination-deaths/11378494

5

M Clarke, 'Anatomy of an epidemic: How measles took hold of Samoa', *ABC News*, 9 December 2019, accessed 21 January 2021. https://www.abc.net.au/news/2019-12-09/anatomy-of-an-epidemic:-how-measles-took-hold-of-samoa/11773018?nw=0

6

AT Craig, AE Heywood, H Worth, 'Measles epidemic in Samoa and other Pacific islands', *The Lancet Infectious Diseases*, 2020, 20(3), 273–275. https://doi.org/10.1016/S1473-3099(20)30053-0

7

A Taylor, 'There was an effective vaccine. An outbreak struck anyway', *The Washington Post*, 7 July 2020, accessed 21 January 2021. https://www.washingtonpost.com/world/2020/07/07/coronavirus-measles-samoa-vaccine/

8

K Gibney, 'Measles in Samoa: How a small island nation found itself in the grips of an outbreak disaster', *The Conversation*, 12 December 2019, accessed 21 January 2021. https://theconversation.com/measles-in-samoa-how-a-small-island-nation-found-itself-in-the-grips-of-an-outbreak-disaster-128467

9

T Winterstein, 'State of Emergency declared and mandatory MMR vaccination for all, starting from 6 months of age ...' Instagram post, 16 November 2019, accessed 21 January 2021.

10

Agence France-Presse, 'Samoa measles outbreak: WHO blames anti-vaccine scare as death toll hits 39', *The Guardian*, 28 November 2019, accessed 21 January 2021. https://www.theguardian.com/world/2019/nov/28/samoa-measles-outbreak-who-blames-anti-vaccine-scare-death-toll?CMP=share_btn_tw

11

F Kerr, 'Samoa measles outbreak: Death toll rises to 44 and is expected to climb further', *Stuff*, 30 November 2019, accessed 21 January 2021. https://www.stuff.co.nz/national/health/117825133/samoa-measles-outbreak-death-toll-rises-to-44-and-is-expected-to-climb-further

12

A Phillips, M Hickie, J Totterdell, J Brotherton, A Dey, R Hill, T Snelling, K Macartney, 'Adverse events following HPV vaccination: 11 years of surveillance in Australia', *Vaccine*, 2020, 38(38), 6038–6046. https://doi.org/10.1016/j.vaccine.2020.06.039

13

MT Hall, KT Simms, J-B Lew, MA Smith, JML Brotherton, M Saville, IH Frazer, K Canfell, 'The projected timeframe until cervical cancer elimination in Australia: A modelling study', *The Lancet Public Health*, 2018, 4(1), E19–E27. https://doi.org/10.1016/S2468-2667(18)30183-X

14

KT Simms, SJB Hanley, MA Smith, A Keane, K Canfell, 'Impact of HPV vaccine hesitancy on cervical cancer in Japan: A modelling study', *The Lancet Public Health*, 2020, 5(4), E223–E234. https://doi.org/10.1016/S2468-2667(20)30010-4

15

'Myths and Realities: Responding to arguments against vaccination',
Australian Government Department of Health and Ageing, May
2013, accessed 21 January 2021. https://www.health.gov.au/sites/
default/files/full-publication-myths-and-realities-5th-ed-2013.pdf

CHAPTER 14: COOKED

1

P Kalina, 'The ratings reality show: The most watched TV of 2013',
The Sydney Morning Herald, 5 December 2013, accessed 21
January 2021. https://www.smh.com.au/entertainment/tv-and-radio/
the-ratings-reality-show-the-most-watched-tv-of-2013-20131204-
2ypc6.html

D Knox, 'Logie Awards 2014: Winners', *TV Tonight*, 27 April 2014,
accessed 21 January 2021. https://tvtonight.com.au/2014/04/logie-
awards-2014-winners.html

2

P Evans, 'My Day on a Plate', *Sunday Life*, 4 November 2012.

P Starke, 'Social media buzzing with talk of activated almonds', news.
com.au, 5 November 2012, accessed 21 January 2021. https://
www.news.com.au/lifestyle/food/activated-almonds-line-lights-up-
twittersphere/news-story/34f25c3167e842b8e389486d1153c201

3

A Harris, S Duck, '*My Kitchen Rules* chef Pete Evans backs extreme
anti-fluoride group', *The Daily Telegraph*, 6 December 2014, accessed
21 January 2021. https://www.dailytelegraph.com.au/news/nsw/
my-kitchen-rules-chef-pete-evans-backs-extreme-antifluoride-group/
news-story/5251ed358cc50721b5122a7b363280e3

4

A Harris, S Duck, '*My Kitchen Rules* chef Pete Evans backs extreme
anti-fluoride group', *The Daily Telegraph*, 6 December 2014, accessed
21 January 2021. https://www.dailytelegraph.com.au/news/nsw/
my-kitchen-rules-chef-pete-evans-backs-extreme-antifluoride-group/
news-story/5251ed358cc50721b5122a7b363280e3

5

M Hopcraft, 'Pete Evans' defence an "abject disappointment"', *The Sydney Morning Herald*, 27 March 2017, accessed 21 January 2021. https://www.smh.com.au/opinion/pete-evans-defence-an-abject-disappointment-20170327-gv7c15.html

6

Australian Government National Health and Medical Research Council, 'NHMRC Public Statement 2017: Water fluoridation and human health in Australia', 2017, accessed 21 January 2021. https://www.nhmrc.gov.au/sites/default/files/documents/reports/fluoridation-public-statement.pdf

7

Australian Government National Health and Medical Research Council, 'NHMRC Public Statement 2017: Water fluoridation and human health in Australia', 2017, accessed 21 January 2021. https://www.nhmrc.gov.au/sites/default/files/documents/reports/fluoridation-public-statement.pdf

8

Dietitians Association of Australia, 'Media Alert: Bubba Yum Yum', 13 March 2015, accessed 21 January 2021. https://dietitiansaustralia.org.au/wp-content/uploads/2017/01/Media-alert-Bubba-Yum-Yum_FINAL.pdf

9

Australian Government National Health and Medical Research Council, 'Eat for Health: Infant Feeding Guidelines', December 2021, accessed 15 February 2021. https://www.eatforhealth.gov.au/sites/default/files/files/the_guidelines/n56_infant_feeding_guidelines_160822(1).pdf

10

I Brennan, 'Pete Evans' co-authored paleo diet cookbook for babies under investigation', *ABC News*, 12 March 2015, accessed 21 January 2021. https://www.abc.net.au/news/2015-03-12/paleo-diet-cookbook-for-babies-under-investigation-pete-evans/6309452

11

C Weaver, 'Exclusive: Pete Evans' cookbook recalled over "dangerous" Paleo baby formula recipe', *The Australian Women's Weekly*, 11

March 2015, accessed 21 January 2021. https://www.nowtolove.com. au/health/diet-nutrition/pete-evans-paleo-diet-book-for-babies-facing-ban-over-public-health-fears-12722

12

S Molloy, 'Moment Pete Evans started to cause a stir', *The Queensland Times*, 8 May 2020, accessed 21 January 2021. https://www.qt.com. au/news/moment-pete-evans-started-to-cause-a-stir/4011726/

13

L Malpass, 'Chef Pete Evans to self-publish baby paleo book', *The Sydney Morning Herald*, 17 March 2015. https://www.smh.com. au/lifestyle/health-and-wellness/chef-pete-evans-to-selfpublish-baby-paleo-book-20150317-1m0ppx.html

14

Dietitians Association of Australia, 'Media Alert: Parents cautioned on new Bubba Yum Yum baby "brew"', 24 April 2015, accessed 21 January 2021. https://dietitiansaustralia.org.au/wp-content/uploads/2017/01/Dietitians-Association-of-Australia-Media-alert-Bubba-Yum-Yum-24-April.pdf

15

'Pete Evans says sunscreen is full of poisonous chemicals – what do the experts have to say?', *ABC News*, 11 July 2016, accessed 21 January 2021, https://www.abc.net.au/news/2016-07-11/pete-evans-says-sunscreen-is-poisonous/7585050

16

A Colangelo, 'Cancer Council slams Pete Evans' sunscreen claim', *The New Daily*, 10 July 2016, accessed 21 January 2021. https://thenewdaily.com.au/life/wellbeing/2016/07/10/pete-evans-sunscreen/

17

Cancer Council Australia, 'Skin Cancer statistics and issues: skin cancer incidence and mortality', 27 October 2020, accessed 21 January 2021. https://wiki.cancer.org.au/skincancerstats/Skin_cancer_incidence_and_mortality

18

'Australian Cancer Incidence and Mortality (ACIM)', Australian Institute of Health and Welfare, 13 September 2019, accessed 16 February

2021. https://ncci.canceraustralia.gov.au/diagnosis/cancer-incidence/
cancer-incidence

19

P Evans, 'Everyday I love to immerse myself in an experience within ...'
Instagram post, 17 December 2018, accessed 16 February 2021.

20

A Sheemar, B Takkar, S Temkar, P Venkatesh, 'Solar retinopathy: the
yellow dot and the rising sun', *The British Medical Journal Case
Reports*, 2017, http://dx.doi.org/10.1136/bcr-2017-222690.

21

Australian Government, 'Elective surgery waiting times 2017-2018',
Australian Institute of Health and Welfare (AIHW), 1 March 2019,
accessed 21 January 2021. https://www.aihw.gov.au/reports/hospitals/
elective-surgery-waiting-times-17-18/contents/summary

22

Australian Government, 'Osteoporosis', Australian Institute of
Health and Welfare, 25 August 2020, accessed 21 January 2021.
https://www.aihw.gov.au/reports/chronic-musculoskeletal-conditions/
osteoporosis/contents/what-is-osteoporosis

23

A Hoh, 'Pete Evans claims dairy removes calcium from bones: What do
the doctors say?', *ABC News*, 29 August 2016, accessed 21 January
2021. abc.net.au/news/2016-08-29/how-important-is-calcium-
doctors-have-their-say-pete-evans/7794132

24

M Ward, '"Questions that need to be asked": Pete Evans endorses
anti-vaxxer', *The Sydney Morning Herald*, 14 March 2019, accessed
21 January 2021. https://www.smh.com.au/lifestyle/health-and-
wellness/questions-that-need-to-be-asked-pete-evans-endorses-anti-
vaxxer-20190314-p5144h.html

25

L Martin, 'Doctors warn Pete Evans to stick to cooking after sharing
anti-vaxx podcast', *The Guardian*, 14 March 2019, accessed 21
January 2021. https://www.theguardian.com/society/2019/mar/14/

doctors-warns-pete-evans-to-stick-to-cooking-after-sharing-anti-vaxx-podcast

26

RMIT ABC Fact Check, 'Pete Evans spruiks a bogus COVID-19 treatment, and other coronavirus misinformation', *ABC News*, 26 April 2020, accessed 21 January 2021. https://www.abc. net.au/news/2020-04-26/pete-evans-coronavirus-biocharger-coronacheck/12173738

27

Australian Government, 'Pete Evans' company fined for alleged COVID-19 advertising breaches', Department of Health, Therapeutic Goods Administration, 24 April 2020, accessed 21 January 2021. https://www.tga.gov.au/media-release/pete-evans-company-fined-alleged-covid-19-advertising-breaches

28

R Conaghan, 'Pete Evans goes off the deep end, is now sharing completely bonkers conspiracy theories', *Junkee*, 12 May 2020, accessed 21 January 2021. https://junkee.com/pete-evans-qanon/253541

29

C Wilson, 'Pete Evans is now posting neo-Nazi symbols and the far-right love it', *Gizmodo*, 17 November 2020, accessed 21 January 2021. https://www.gizmodo.com.au/2020/11/pete-evans-is-now-posting-neo-nazi-symbols-and-the-far-right-love-it/

30

A Meade, 'Pete Evans dumped by Channel Ten, Coles and Woolworths after posting neo-Nazi symbol', *The Guardian*, 17 November 2020, accessed 21 January 2021. https://www.theguardian.com/australia-news/2020/nov/17/pete-evans-dumped-by-channel-ten-coles-and-woolworths-after-posting-neo-nazi-symbol

CHAPTER 15: THE COVID-19 CONSPIRACY

1

K Corcoran, 'An infamous WHO tweet saying there was "no clear evidence" COVID-19 could spread between humans was posted for "balance" to reflect findings from China', *Business Insider Australia*, 18 April 2020, accessed 21 January 2021. https://www.businessinsider.com.au/who-no-transmission-coronavirus-tweet-was-to-appease-china-guardian-2020-4?r=US&IR=T

2

'Scott Morrison defends decision to attend rugby league game during coronavirus outbreak' [video], *The Guardian*, 13 March 2020, accessed 21 January 2021. https://www.theguardian.com/australia-news/video/2020/mar/13/scott-morrison-defends-decision-to-attend-rugby-league-game-during-coronavirus-outbreak-video

'Scott Morrison cancels plans to attend Cronulla Sharks NRL game amid coronavirus fears', *SBS News*, 14 March 2020, accessed 21 January 2021. https://www.sbs.com.au/news/scott-morrison-cancels-plans-to-attend-cronulla-sharks-nrl-game-amid-coronavirus-fears

3

L Wamsley, 'IMAGES: What new coronavirus looks like under the microscope', *NPR*, 13 February 2020, accessed 21 January 2021. https://www.npr.org/2020/02/13/805837103/images-what-new-coronavirus-looks-like-under-the-microscope

4

A Camerota, J Doering, 'Nurse: Some patients who test positive refuse to believe they have COVID-19' [video], *CNN*, 16 November 2020, accessed 21 January 2021. https://edition.cnn.com/videos/us/2020/11/16/south-dakota-nurse-intv-newday-vpx.cnn/video/playlists/new-day-highlights/

5

R Heilweil, 'How the 5G coronavirus conspiracy theory went from fringe to mainstream', *Vox*, 24 April 2020, accessed 21 January 2021. https://www.vox.com/recode/2020/4/24/21231085/coronavirus-5g-conspiracy-theory-covid-facebook-youtube

S Nicholls, A Russell, N Selvaratnam, 'What is the truth about 5G? Four Corners spoke to leading experts and anti-5G activists to find out', *ABC News*, 3 August 2020, accessed 21 January 2021. https://www.abc.net.au/news/2020-08-03/5g-conspiracy-theory-investigation-coronavirus-health/12507368

6

IA Hamilton, '77 cell phone towers have been set on fire so far due to a weird coronavirus 5G conspiracy theory', *Business Insider,* 7 May 2020, accessed 21 January 2021. https://www.businessinsider.com.au/77-phone-masts-fire-coronavirus-5g-conspiracy-theory-2020-5?r=US&IR=T

7

World Health Organization, 'Coronavirus disease (COVID-19) advice for the public: Mythbusters', 23 November 2020, accessed 21 January 2021. https://www.who.int/emergencies/diseases/novel-coronavirus-2019/advice-for-public/myth-busters

8

'Lorna Jane fined almost $40,000 for alleged advertising breaches in relation to COVID-19 and "anti-virus activewear"', Australian Government, Department of Health Therapeutic Goods Administration, 17 July 2020, accessed 21 January 2021. https://www.tga.gov.au/media-release/lorna-jane-fined-almost-40000-alleged-advertising-breaches-relation-covid-19-and-anti-virus-activewear

9

MS Islam, T Sarkar, SH Khan, A-H Mostofa Kamal, SM Murshid Hasan, A Kabir, D Yeasmin, MA Islam, KI Amin Chowdhury, KS Anwar, AA Chughtai, H Seale, 'COVID-19-related infodemic and its impact on public health: A global social media analysis', *The American Journal of Tropical Medicine and Hygiene*, 2020, 103(4), 1621–1629. https://doi.org/10.4269/ajtmh.20-0812

10

A Yussuf, 'Clive Palmer has bought 30 million doses of an anti-malaria drug to fight COVID-19. But experts warn this may not be the cure-all', *The Feed SBS*, 29 April 2020, accessed 21 January 2021. https://www.sbs.com.au/news/the-feed/clive-palmer-has-bought-30-million-doses-of-an-anti-malaria-drug-to-fight-covid-19-but-experts-warn-this-may-not-be-the-cure-all

P Karp, 'Liberal MP Craig Kelly's hydroxychloroquine claims should be removed from social media, regulator says', *The Guardian*,

16 September 2020, accessed 21 January 2021. https://www.
theguardian.com/media/2020/sep/16/liberal-mp-craig-kellys-
hydroxychloroquine-claims-should-be-removed-from-social-media-
regulator-says

CHAPTER 16: FIXING THE FUTURE

1

G Dixon, C Clarke, 'The effect of falsely balanced reporting of the
autism-vaccine controversy on vaccine safety perceptions and
behavioral intentions', Health Education Research, 2013, 28(2),
352–359. https://doi.org/10.1093/her/cys110

R Dunlop, 'Anti-vaccination activists should not be given a say in the
media', *The Guardian*, 16 October 2013, accessed 21 January 2021.
https://www.theguardian.com/commentisfree/2013/oct/16/anti-
vaccination-activists-should-not-be-given-a-say-in-the-media

2

D Wolfe, D Dale, '"It's going to disappear": a timeline of Trump's claims
that COVID-19 will vanish', *CNN*, 31 October 2020, accessed
21 January 2021. https://edition.cnn.com/interactive/2020/10/politics/
covid-disappearing-trump-comment-tracker/

3

J Henley, 'How Finland starts its fight against fake news in primary
schools', *The Guardian*, 29 January 2020, accessed 21 January 2021.
https://www.theguardian.com/world/2020/jan/28/fact-from-fiction-
finlands-new-lessons-in-combating-fake-news

4

E Mackintosh, E Kiernan, 'Finland is winning the war on fake news.
What it's learned may be crucial to Western democracy', *CNN*,
May 2019, accessed 21 January 2021. https://edition.cnn.com/
interactive/2019/05/europe/finland-fake-news-intl/

hachette
AUSTRALIA

If you would like to find out more about Hachette Australia, our authors, upcoming events and new releases you can visit our website or our social media channels:

hachette.com.au

f HachetteAustralia

𝕏 📷 HachetteAus